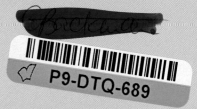
THE

Arthritis Foundation's

guide to

Managing Your

ARTHRITIS

MARY ANNE DUNKIN

Chief Medical Editor
John H. Klippel, MD

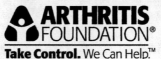
AN OFFICIAL PUBLICATION
OF THE ARTHRITIS FOUNDATION

ABOUT THE AUTHOR

Mary Anne Dunkin is an experienced journalist specializing in arthritis and related diseases, and other medical topics. She served as Senior Editor for *Arthritis Today* magazine for six years, and currently works as a contributing editor to the magazine. Ms. Dunkin and her family live in suburban Atlanta. This is her first book.

ACKNOWLEDGMENTS

The Arthritis Foundation's Guide to Managing Your Arthritis is written for people who have arthritis or other related diseases, as well as for their friends, family and loved ones. Bringing this book to completion was a team effort, including the significant contributions of dedicated physicians, health-care professionals, Arthritis Foundation volunteers, writers, editors, designers and Arthritis Foundation staff.

Special acknowledgments should go to Mary Anne Dunkin, the author of the book. The chief medical editor of the book was John H. Klippel, MD, the Medical Director of the Arthritis Foundation. The book was reviewed by James R. O'Dell, MD, of the Department of Internal Medicine at the University of Nebraska Medical Center in Omaha; Lee S. Simon, MD, of the Department of Medicine at Beth Israel Deaconness Medical Center in Boston; and E. William St. Clair, MD, of the Department of Medicine at Duke University Medical Center in Durham, NC. The author would also like to thank Doyt Conn, MD, Professor of Medicine, Director of Allergy, Immunology and Rheumatology at Emory University School of Medicine in Atlanta, for his guidance during the writing of this book.

The editorial director of the book is Susan Bernstein. The art director is Susan Siracusa. Layout production was done by Darryl Moland.

All Arthritis Foundation books are available through our fulfillment center order line, 1-800-207-8633, or on the Arthritis Foundation Web site, **www.arthritis.org.** Arthritis Foundation books are also available in fine retail bookstores.

A FEW WORDS ABOUT THE ARTHRITIS FOUNDATION

The Arthritis Foundation is the only nationwide, nonprofit health organization helping people take greater control of arthritis by leading efforts to prevent, control and cure arthritis and related diseases – the nation's number one cause of disability. Nearly 43 million Americans currently have arthritis or a related condition – and that number is expected to grow in the coming years. To serve this population, Arthritis Foundation volunteers and staff nationwide provide information, programs, services and research assistance.

The Arthritis Foundation's efforts center on the three-fold mission of the organization: research, prevention and quality of life. The Arthritis Foundation currently provides more than $20 million in grants to more than 300 researchers to help find a cure, prevention or better treatment for arthritis. The Arthritis Foundation's sponsorship of research for more than 50 years has resulted in major treatment advances for most arthritis-related diseases. You will learn more about these diseases and their many treatments in this book.

The Arthritis Foundation, which has more than 150 chapters and branch offices to serve people with arthritis in communities nationwide, provides a number of community-based programs and services. More information about these offerings are included in the resources section at the end of this book. In addition, Arthritis Foundation volunteers serve as advocates to local and national governments on behalf of people with arthritis. Their successes include the federal establishment of a national institute for arthritis among the National Institutes of Health, increased federal funding for arthritis research and state funding for arthritis medications. The Arthritis Foundation has an array of award-winning publications, including the bimonthly magazine *Arthritis Today*; a number of books, brochures and subscription newsletters; and an interactive Web site, **www.arthritis.org**, which offers a wealth of information about arthritis, current research and advocacy-related news, and an interactive self-management program, *Connect and Control*.

To learn more about membership in the Arthritis Foundation, which includes a subscription to *Arthritis Today*, or the programs and services available in your area, contact your local chapter by calling 800/283-7800, or log on to **www.arthritis.org.**

Contents

Contents *continued*

FOREWORD

Arthritis is one of the most common diseases affecting Americans today – nearly 43 million people in this country live with some form of arthritis. Arthritis strikes people of all ages, including children, and over the next two decades, the number of people with arthritis is expected to increase to as many as 60 million people. Arthritis is not just one disease, but more than 100 different disorders that affect joints, muscles, tendons, and in many instances internal organs of the body. All forms of arthritis impact people's lives in profound ways ranging from the limited activities caused by pain or inability to fully use a joint affected by arthritis, to severe and even life-threatening complications associated with many forms of arthritis.

There are four key steps for successful treatment of all forms of arthritis. First, learn as much as you can about arthritis and treatment options available to you. Second, make a decision to do something about the arthritis. Third, see a doctor to learn what type of arthritis you have. Finally, work with your doctor to develop a plan of treatment.

Arthritis treatment is very much dependent on the type of arthritis being treated. For example, osteoarthritis (the most common form of arthritis) is treated very differently from rheumatoid arthritis, lupus or fibromyalgia. Moreover, most forms of arthritis are chronic. Treatment needs and goals typically change over time, and require a close working relationship between the person with arthritis, their doctor, and other members of a health-care team for success of the treatment.

There are now a number of very effective approaches available for the person with arthritis. Regular exercise, weight control and avoiding injury to joints are important for essentially all forms of arthritis, particularly osteoarthritis. Medications, including both over-the-counter and prescription drugs, play an important role in pain management. Over the past decade, there have been major advances in new medicines available for arthritis treatment. In addition, there has been a tremendous interest and increase in the use of alternative or complementary medicines for arthritis. Finally, surgery to replace joints irreversibly damaged by arthritis has become an almost routine procedure when a person's arthritis has made them practically immobile.

This book, *The Arthritis Foundation's Guide to Managing Your Arthritis*, gives you the tools you will need to understand your arthritis treatment and to take control to more effectively manage your arthritis. In these pages, you will learn about the most common forms of arthritis, their many symptoms, how your doctor will diagnose your disease and how you will work with your health-care professional to begin a course of treatment. You will learn about the many drugs, surgical therapies and alternative approaches to treating arthritis. Most importantly, you will learn how your actions will impact your health – from exercise to diet to stress and pain management. This book will help you take control of arthritis – instead of allowing arthritis to take control of your life.

The Arthritis Foundation believes that the actions taken by people with arthritis play a large and important role in determining their outcome. Education, self-management, and taking personal responsibility are tools of empowerment and keys to achieving control of arthritis. *The Arthritis Foundation's Guide to Managing Your Arthritis* is a practical and clear guide that will help you achieve a healthier, more fulfilling life with arthritis.

John H. Klippel, MD
Medical Director
Arthritis Foundation
Atlanta, GA

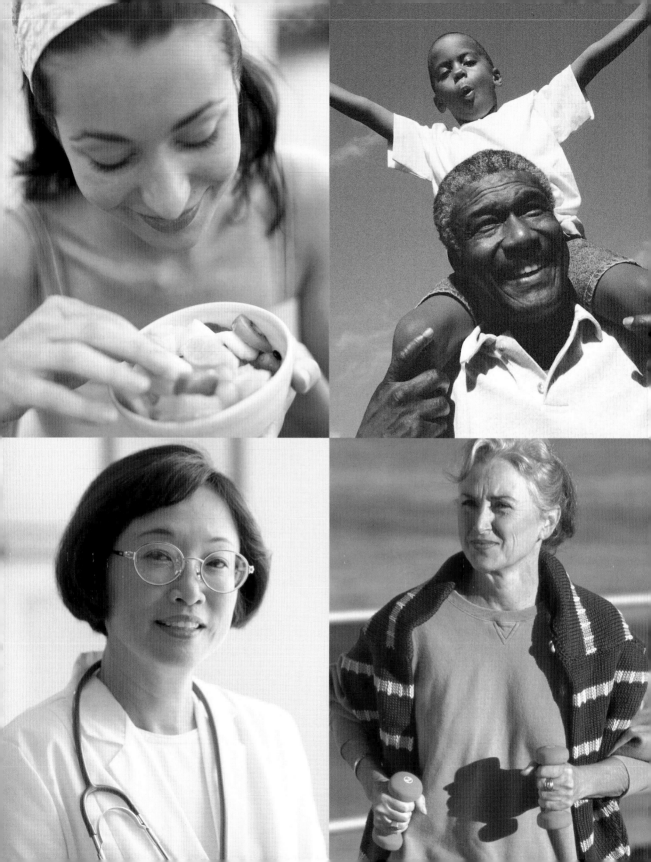

Introduction

You probably are reading this book because you or someone you love has arthritis. You're not alone. Arthritis is one of the most common medical conditions affecting Americans, and as the population ages, the numbers of people affected by arthritis are only going to increase. At the time of this book's publication, an estimated 43 million Americans have some form of arthritis or a related disease. If predictions by the Centers for Disease Control and Prevention hold true, this number will rise to nearly 60 million Americans by the year 2020.

Although the prevalence of certain forms of arthritis increases with age, arthritis is not just a disease of older people. In fact, arthritis is not a disease at all, but a term used to refer to more than 100 related conditions that can cause pain, stiffness, swelling, inflammation and damage to joints and surrounding tissues. Arthritis in its various forms can affect anyone of any age, causing altered growth, school and work absences, and difficulty performing basic daily tasks.

But the prognosis is not all bleak – far from it! Proper treatment can relieve pain and other symptoms and, in some cases, slow or halt the disease process. Never before have physicians had so many options to offer people with arthritis, and advances in treatment are occurring at an unprecedented pace.

In the past, many people with arthritis believed that their role in treatment was passive. They believed that there was little they could do except take the medications their doctor prescribed, have surgery if necessary and learn to live with the pain, stiffness, limited mobility and other symptoms associated with their disease. This passive role left them feeling out of control, and often allowed arthritis to take over their lives.

Now, when people are first diagnosed with arthritis, their physicians tell them that the most important thing a person with a chronic illness must do is take control. People with arthritis must take an active role in their treatment, a practice known as *self-management*. Self-managers work with their rheumatologists and other health-care professionals in a partnership of care, asking questions, keeping track of pain and other symptoms, engaging in healthy lifestyle practices and exploring various options for treatment. Self-management includes taking an active role while you are in the doctor's office as well as in daily life.

In addition to faithfully taking the medications your doctor prescribes – and alerting him to medication-related problems – you can take many measures to ease your symptoms and live well with arthritis. These methods cover a wide range, from exercise and proper diet to mind-body techniques that reduce pain and stress. In this book, you'll learn the basics for many of these methods and techniques. You will learn important information about the causes and symptoms of arthritis, the most common arthritis drugs and surgical therapies, and self-management strategies that will help you control pain and other problems. Although you may need the help of a professional to get you started, you can take control of your treatment.

Whether you are new to arthritis or have lived with it for years, this book should have something to help you. You'll find information for every step of your journey with arthritis, from getting a diagnosis to assembling a health-care team to evaluating arthritis information on the Internet to recuperating from surgery, if that action is necessary. Let this book challenge you to learn more about your condition, open the lines of communication with your physician, work in partnership with your health-care team and take steps to find out what works for you.

The concept of being responsible for managing your arthritis may seem overwhelming at first, especially if you were raised in an era when patients unquestioningly followed doctors' orders. With some practical advice, encouragement and a little time, the concept can be liberating. You can do something about your arthritis, and this book is a great way to get started.

PART ONE

UNDERSTANDING ARTHRITIS

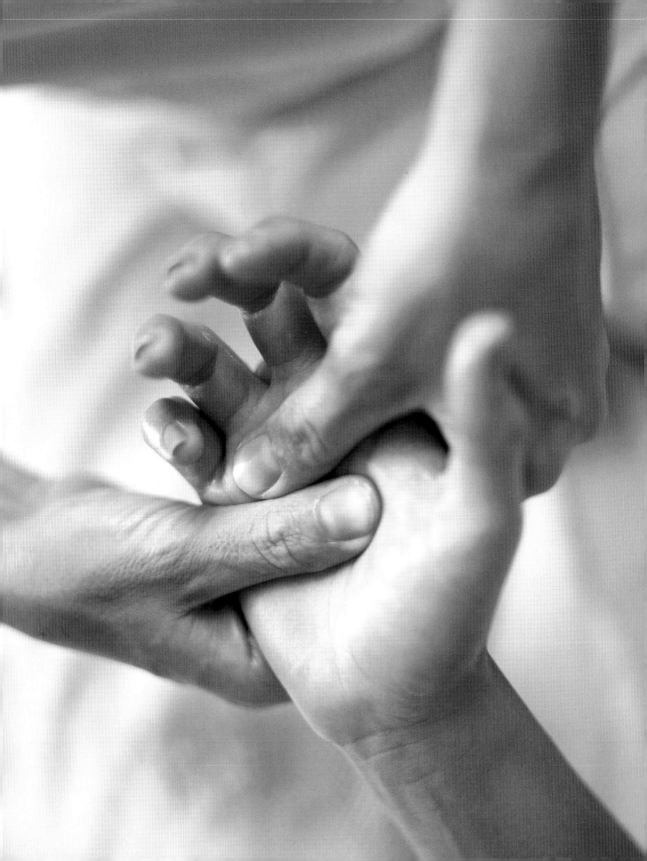

What Is Arthritis?

1

CHAPTER 1: WHAT IS ARTHRITIS?

Mention the word arthritis and many people think of the aches and pains that occur naturally with age. If you have arthritis yourself, you probably know all too well that it's much more than aches and pains, there's nothing natural about it, and you don't have to be old to have it. Furthermore, arthritis technically is not an "it," but a whole collection of related diseases.

While often referred to as if it were a single disease, arthritis is actually an umbrella term used for a group of more than 100 medical conditions that collectively affect nearly 43 million Americans of all ages. While the most common form of arthritis – osteoarthritis (OA) – is most prevalent in people over age 60, arthritis in its various forms can start as early as infancy. Some forms affect people in their young-adult years as they are beginning careers and families and still others start during the peak career and child-rearing years.

The common thread among these 100-plus conditions is that they all affect the musculo-skeletal system and specifically the *joints* – where two or more bones meet (see diagrams below). Arthritis-related joint problems include pain, stiffness, inflammation and damage to joint cartilage (the tough, smooth tissue that covers the ends of the bones, enabling them to glide against one another) and surrounding structures. Such damage can lead to joint weakness, instability and visible deformities that, depending on the location of joint involvement, can interfere with the most basic daily tasks such as walking, climbing stairs, using a computer keyboard, cutting your food or brushing your teeth.

For many people with arthritis, however, joint involvement is not the extent of the problem.

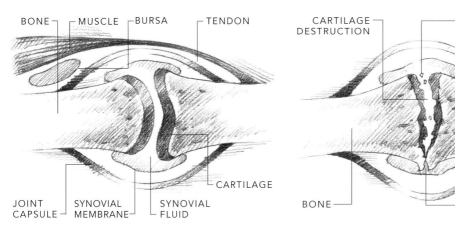

BONE — MUSCLE — BURSA — TENDON
CARTILAGE DESTRUCTION — LOOSE CARTILAGE PARTICLES

JOINT CAPSULE — SYNOVIAL MEMBRANE — SYNOVIAL FLUID — CARTILAGE
BONE — BONE SPUR

A NORMAL JOINT — A JOINT WITH OSTEOARTHRITIS

WHAT IS A JOINT?

The joints, which link our 206 bones, are among the body's most ingenious structures and make almost any type of movement possible.

Some joints, such as the elbows and knees, are called hinge joints. They move back and forth like an opening and closing door. Ball-and-socket joints, such as the hip or shoulder, enable bones to twist and turn in many directions while staying firmly connected to each other. Other joints, such as those of the pelvis, move little, and some, such as the joints of the skull, where rigidity is desirable, don't move at all.

Despite their many marvels, joints have their limits. While they thrive with use, excess use can be harmful. They are also subject to damage – either through trauma or any of the 100-plus forms of arthritis. In understanding arthritis, it helps to have a basic knowledge of what a joint is and the structures that make up a joint.

Basically, a joint is where two or more bones meet. Our bodies have close to 150 of those junctures. Covering the ends of those bones is a smooth, rubbery tissue called *cartilage* that acts as a shock absorber and allows the joint to move smoothly. Some joints are cushioned by small, fluid-filled sacs, called *bursae*. The entire joint is enclosed in capsule composed of tough connective tissue and lined with a thin membrane called the *synovium*. The synovium secretes a viscous, or slippery, liquid called synovial fluid. That fluid lubricates the joints, making movement easier.

Surrounding and supporting your joints are soft tissues, including *muscles*, which are made up of stretchable fibers that help move parts of the body; *tendons*, which are fibers at the ends of muscles that connect them to the bones; and *ligaments*, which are supporting tissues that attach to bones and help keep them together at a joint.

Depending on the particular form of arthritis you have, almost any of these structures – from the cartilage and synovium inside the joint to the ligaments and tendons that support the joint – can be affected.

Many forms of arthritis are classified as *systemic*, meaning they can affect the whole body. In these diseases, arthritis can cause damage to virtually any bodily organ or system, including the heart, lungs, kidneys, blood vessels and skin. Arthritis-related conditions primarily affect the muscles and bones.

Together, arthritis and related conditions are a major cause of disability in the United States, costing the U.S. economy nearly $65 billion per year in medical care and indirect expenses such as lost wages and production – and costing millions of individuals their health, their physical abilities and, in many cases, their independence. And unless something changes, the picture is going to get worse. As the population ages, the number of people with arthritis is growing.

There is good news for people with arthritis. Things are changing. While the number of people with arthritis is increasing, in general, these people are faring better than at any time in history. While there is currently no cure for arthritis, most forms can be managed successfully with available medication and non-medication treatments. In the meantime, research is leading to a better understanding of arthritis-related diseases, better ways to diagnose them and more, better and safer treatments for them.

Research is also helping to identify genes involved in different forms of arthritis. For example, a decade ago, researchers found a gene mutation that was responsible for a defect in type II collagen, a major component of joint cartilage. The gene mutation, they found, ran in families and caused defective cartilage that is prone to breakdown. As a result, people with the mutation developed premature osteoarthritis – often by their 20s.

While the link between genes and other forms of arthritis is less clear, most arthritis-related diseases – if not all – are believed to have a genetic component. In many of them, genetic markers have been identified. But that doesn't mean that you will develop a certain form of arthritis just because a parent, sibling, aunt or uncle has it. It is likely that a number of genes, along with other factors such as a virus, bacterium or something else in the environment, cause the development of arthritis in certain people.

By identifying and better understanding the involved genes, doctors hope not only to create better treatments for arthritis, but to be able to target treatment at people with the greatest risk of severe disease. The hope is that early, aggressive treatment in combination with lifestyle modifications (such as losing excess pounds or limiting activities that would put undue stress on arthritis-susceptible joints) may help minimize or even prevent some types of arthritis-related joint damage.

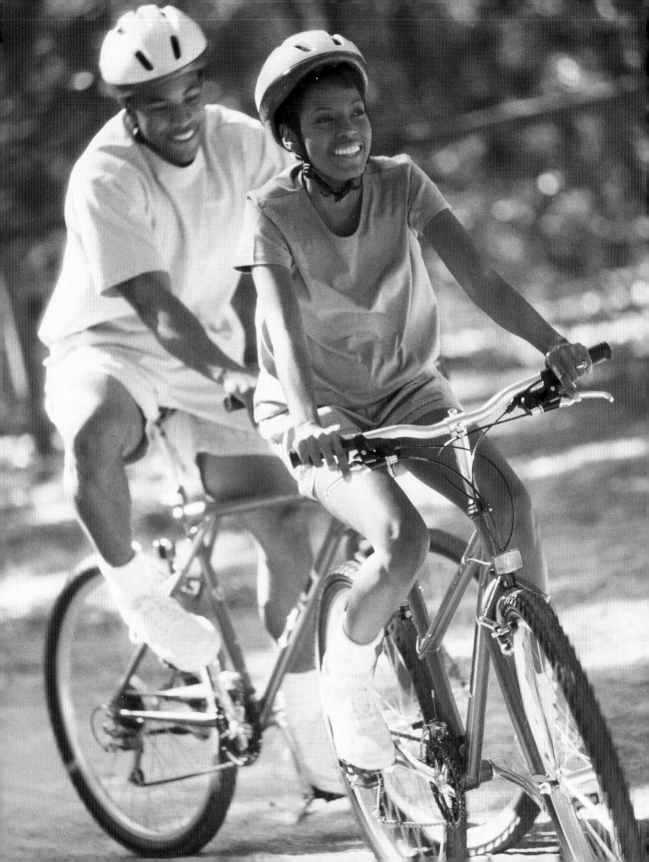

What Kind of Arthritis Do I Have?

2

CHAPTER 2: WHAT KIND OF ARTHRITIS DO I HAVE?

If you have experienced joint pain, stiffness, swelling or inflammation, you may have arthritis. You probably picked up this book because you suspect that you or someone you love has arthritis. But what type of arthritis could it be?

As discussed, arthritis is not a single disease, although the term often is used as if it is one disease. Instead, arthritis refers to more than 100 different forms of the disease and related conditions. The similarity among the different forms is that they affect the joints, generally causing pain. Arthritis and related conditions may cause pain and damage to the connective tissue of the muscles, ligaments, tendons, bones, skin and internal organs.

Discussing all of the different forms of arthritis and related conditions is beyond the scope of this book, and most forms of the disease are quite rare. In this chapter, you'll learn about some of the most common forms and related conditions. You may think you recognize your condition from these descriptions, and you may be right. But arthritis cannot be diagnosed by reading a book. If you don't have a diagnosis from a physician, it's important that you see one. Different forms of arthritis usually are treated differently; you may need to see a *rheumatologist* (a doctor who specializes in arthritis) to get the specialized care you need. Ultimately,

prompt and proper treatment offers the best chance to prevent damage and complications of the disease.

OSTEOARTHRITIS

Osteoarthritis (OA), the most common form of arthritis, affects 21 million people. Although it grows increasingly common and often painful with age, an estimated 12.1 percent of Americans aged 25 and older have clinical signs and symptoms of OA. Like many other forms of arthritis, it is more common in women than in men.

If you have osteoarthritis, you probably experience morning stiffness and mild to moderate

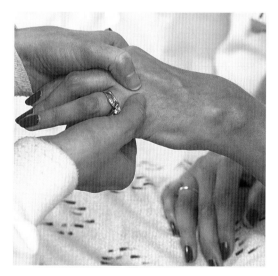

pain that may come on slowly throughout the day or may come and go periodically. On the other hand, you may have pain and stiffness that steadily worsen, making it difficult to go about your daily life.

The pain of OA usually is in or around the affected joints, which most commonly are joints of the knees, hips, fingers, neck and lower back. Knuckles, wrists, elbows, shoulders and ankles are affected very rarely. If osteoarthritic joint changes cause pressure on the nerves and muscles surrounding the joint, the pain may be felt elsewhere, a problem known as referred pain. For example, osteoarthritis in the neck may be felt as pain in the shoulder.

Deformities due to overgrowth of bone at the margins of the joint are common in osteoarthritis, particularly in the fingers. Knobby bone growths in the finger joints nearest the nails are called *Heberden's nodes*, and growths in the middle of the fingers are called *Bouchard's nodes*, named for the physicians who first described them (see diagram below.) Such growths tend

to run in families and are more common in women than in men. The nodes may appear on only one finger or on several fingers. They may cause chronic or intermittent pain and interfere with the ability to enjoy such leisure activities as needlework, playing the piano or golfing.

Until recently, osteoarthritis was considered a normal part of the aging process; it was believed that joint cartilage naturally deteriorated after years of use. Increasingly, however, doctors believe that OA is not an inevitable part of aging. They now realize that OA may result from a number of factors, including:

- **Genetic defects in cartilage.** At least one genetic abnormality, a mutation of a gene that codes for Type II collagen, a major component of joint cartilage, has been associated with OA in certain people with premature development of the disease.
- **Congenital abnormalities in joint alignment.** When joints are not aligned properly from birth, the joints can wear irregularly, leading

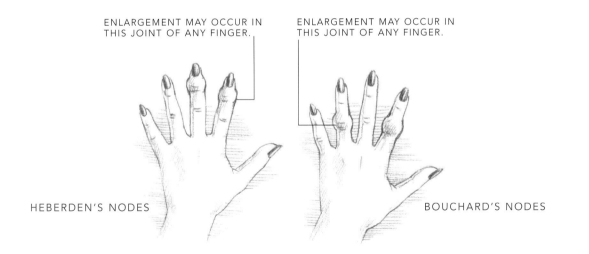

ENLARGEMENT MAY OCCUR IN THIS JOINT OF ANY FINGER.

ENLARGEMENT MAY OCCUR IN THIS JOINT OF ANY FINGER.

HEBERDEN'S NODES

BOUCHARD'S NODES

to OA. Recent studies show that OA of the knee is more common in people with bowed legs or knock knees. People born with shallow hip sockets are likely to develop OA of the hip later in life.

- **Joint injuries that compromise the integrity of the joint.** Like congenital abnormalities, joint injuries that alter joint alignment or stability can lead to irregular wear and osteoarthritis.
- **Overuse of a particular joint.** Excessive use can lead to cartilage wear and OA.
- **Obesity.** The more weight you carry, the larger the load your joints have to support. Excessive weight is recognized as a major risk factor for the development and worsening of osteoarthritis of the knee and probably the hip.

RHEUMATOID ARTHRITIS

The second most common form of arthritis, rheumatoid arthritis (RA), affects an estimated 2.1 million people – 600,000 men and 1.5 million women. Although it can occur in people of any age, most cases are diagnosed in people between the ages of 30 and 50. Rheumatoid arthritis also affects an estimated 30,000 to 50,000 children. (For more information on juvenile rheumatoid arthritis, see the discussion of juvenile arthritis, beginning on the next page.)

The pain of RA is caused by inflammation of the synovium, the thin membrane that lines the joint. Inflammation can be so severe that it damages cartilage, bone and connective tissue.

If you have rheumatoid arthritis, your joints probably are affected in a symmetrical fashion. That is, if one elbow or knee is inflamed and painful, the other elbow or knee likely will be. The joints RA is most likely to affect are those of the fingers, hands, wrists, elbows, shoulders, knees, ankles and feet.

Although no one fully understands RA, generally it is believed to be an *autoimmune disease*. In autoimmune diseases, the body's immune system, which is designed to protect us from such harmful invaders as viruses and bacteria, mistakenly turns against healthy tissue. The joint is the main site of this attack, but RA can affect the entire body. For example, you may run a low-grade fever and experience fatigue and general achiness. In rare cases, RA can affect the skin, muscles and internal organs, such as the heart and lungs.

What causes the immune system to attack healthy tissues is unknown, but scientists suspect an interplay of genetic and environmental factors may be to blame. One genetic marker, HLA-DR4, has been associated with RA development and severity.

Environmental factors suspected of playing a role in the disease include viral or bacterial infections, coffee and cigarette smoke. A recent study showed that older women who smoked were more than twice as likely to have RA as those who never smoked, and other studies have linked smoking to RA severity. A large Finnish study showed that people who drank four or more cups of coffee daily were twice as likely to have *rheumatoid facto*r, an antibody associated with rheumatoid arthritis.

Because RA is approximately three times more common in women than in men, scientists believe that female hormones also may play a role. Interestingly, the use of birth control pills has been shown to offer some protection against the disease. Furthermore, during pregnancy, women who have RA often experience remissions or decreased disease activity. Researchers are trying to better understand the connection between genes, hormones and other factors that play a role in RA. The hope is that a better understanding of these factors will lead to better treatments and, eventually, ways to prevent and cure the disease.

JUVENILE ARTHRITIS

When arthritis begins before age 16, it is classified as juvenile arthritis. Although children can have almost any form of arthritis that adults can have, the most common form in children is juvenile rheumatoid arthritis (JRA), which is further categorized as pauciarticular (affecting four or fewer joints), polyarticular (affecting five or more joints) and systemic (affecting the entire body).

Depending on the type, JRA may be relatively mild, or it can be progressive and disabling; it may be limited to the joints or affect the eyes and other organs. In some cases, JRA resolves by adulthood; in others, its effects are lifelong, requiring ongoing medical care. The number of cases of JRA in the United States is estimated between 30,000 and 50,000.

FIBROMYALGIA

The most common arthritis-related condition, fibromyalgia, affects around four million people, most of them women. Unlike most conditions you'll read about in this book, fibromyalgia does not affect the joints. Instead, fibromyalgia is characterized by widespread pain and fatigue that can be debilitating.

Another common characteristic of fibromyalgia is the presence of *tender points*, or specific areas of the body that are particularly painful upon application of the slightest pressure. Because fibromyalgia can make you feel generally bad all over, many people don't even realize they have these tender points until a doctor presses on them during a physical exam. Yet, tender points are so common in people with fibromyalgia that they are among the primary criteria physicians use to diagnose the condition. (For more information about tender points, see Chapter 3, "Diagnosing Arthritis.")

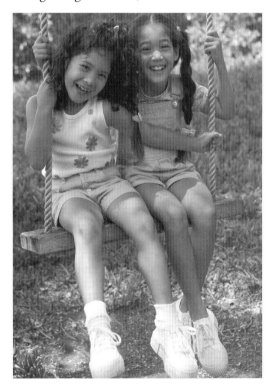

If you have fibromyalgia, you may feel as if you have a never-ending case of the flu or as though you haven't slept for weeks. In fact, you may not have slept – at least, not well. Up to 85 percent of people with fibromyalgia experience problems with sleep. They may fall asleep without difficulty, but they sleep lightly and wake up frequently throughout the night. They often wake up feeling tired, even after sleeping all night.

Other problems associated with fibromyalgia include headaches; difficulty concentrating; frequent constipation or diarrhea, or a combination of the two in conjunction with abdominal pain (a condition known as irritable bowel syndrome); bladder spasms or bladder irritability or urgency (which make you feel as though you always need to go to the bathroom or that you must go immediately); and pain or dysfunction with the temporomandibular joints (TMJ), which attach the lower jaw to the skull on each side of the face.

Although the cause of fibromyalgia is not known, scientists suspect that several factors – including infectious illness, physical or emotional trauma or hormonal changes, alone or in combination – may contribute to the generalized pain, fatigue and sleep disturbances that characterize the condition. Some studies have suggested that people with fibromyalgia have abnormal levels of several chemicals that help transmit and amplify pain signals to and from the brain.

Whether these abnormalities are a cause or result of fibromyalgia is unknown. Because of the prevalence of this condition and the lack of understanding about its causes and optimal treatment, fibromyalgia has become the subject of increased research focus in recent years.

ANKYLOSING SPONDYLITIS

Ankylosing spondylitis (AS) is one of a group of diseases collectively referred to as the *spondyloarthropathies*, a term that means arthritis that affects the spine. In addition to AS, this group of inflammatory diseases includes reactive arthritis, psoriatic arthritis and arthritis with inflammatory bowel disease. Together, the spondyloarthropathies affect an estimated 400,000 people.

The most obvious common characteristic of the spondyloarthropathies, from which they get the name, is their similar effects on the spine. Typically, these diseases attack the *sacroiliac joints* that attach the spine to the pelvis and the stack of bones called vertebrae, which form the spinal column. Other common features include an association between the diseases and a genetic type called HLA-B27; the presence of arthritis in other joints (commonly, the shoulders, hips, knees and ankles); and occasional involvement of other tissues, including those of the skin, eyes, bowel and genitourinary tract.

Traditionally, ankylosing spondylitis was thought to be primarily a disease of young men. However, doctors have begun to realize that AS also affects women – perhaps as often as it does men. However, AS may appear differently in women, and in women, its effects usually are less severe.

If you have ankylosing spondylitis, your symptoms likely began gradually, with lower back pain that you first may have noted at night in bed. As in other forms of arthritis, however, the symptoms can vary greatly from person to person. In some people, AS first shows up as pain or inflammation in such joints as a knee or hip.

In the most severe and advanced cases of AS, the tissues that support the spine can become ossified, or bone-like. When the tissues ossify, the spine may stiffen and fuse in one position, causing the body to lock in a stooped or rigid, upright position. A similar process of ossification in the ligaments that attach the ribs to the spine may make breathing difficult. In some people, AS may affect the eyes, heart and lungs. In the vast majority of people, however, fusion and organ involvement never occur.

Although no one is certain what causes ankylosing spondylitis, the finding of HLA-B27 in most people with the disease leads scientists to believe that there is an inherited component. However, because many people without the disease also have the gene, something else must be involved, such as an environmental factor that triggers the disease in susceptible people. Research in recent years has suggested that normal bowel bacteria may trigger the disease in people who are genetically predisposed to it. Other research is likely to uncover other possible triggers, as well as better ways to treat or even halt the disease.

GOUT

If you go to bed fine and wake up with excruciating pain in a single joint, typically the big toe, you probably have gout, a disease that affects some 2.1 million people nationwide.

Primarily a disease of men, gout rarely is seen in women before menopause. Gout occurs when a bodily waste product called uric acid builds up in the body. Normally, excess uric acid is filtered out by the kidneys. When the kidneys don't eliminate uric acid efficiently, or when the body produces too much of it, the acid can crystallize in joints, causing pain and inflammation.

Gout usually strikes a single joint suddenly. Inflammation and swelling of the affected joint may be so severe that the skin over the joint is pulled taut and appears shiny and red or purplish. Typically, inflammation subsides on its own within a week or so. However, unless the high level of uric acid is treated, attacks will return with increasing frequency and affect more joints, including the feet, knees and elbows. If allowed to progress, gout can lead to joint damage.

Fortunately, gout is well understood, treatable and preventable. Appropriate treatment can reduce the frequency and severity of attacks and may prevent future attacks. (See "The Gout Exception," on page 138.)

LUPUS

Systemic lupus erythematosus (SLE), often referred to simply as lupus, is an inflammatory disease that affects an estimated 250,000 Americans. It affects six times as many women as men and four times as many African Americans as Caucasians. It is most likely to begin during a woman's childbearing years.

Like other forms of arthritis, lupus causes inflammation of the joints, typically those of the hands, wrists, elbows, knees and feet. Because it is a systemic disease, it also can affect the skin, blood, lungs, kidneys and cardiovascular and nervous systems.

If you have lupus, the first symptoms you notice may include fatigue, fever, achiness, weight loss, swollen glands, skin rashes (especially over the cheeks and bridge of the nose) and pain in the joints, chest and abdomen.

Over time, you may experience other signs and symptoms, such as a sensitivity to sunlight that causes rashes after minimal sun exposure; sores on the tongue, inside the mouth and in the nose; chest pain; shortness of breath; swelling of the legs and feet; blanching of the fingers in response to cold temperatures or stress; and dry eyes and mouth.

As the disease progresses, you may experience periods when the disease becomes more active (a flare) or becomes less active or inactive (a remission). On rare occasions, a person may have a complete or long-lasting remission. Like most other forms of arthritis, lupus is chronic, meaning that it lasts a long time – usually a lifetime. However, in most people, lupus becomes less active with age.

Although no one is certain what causes lupus, like rheumatoid arthritis, it is considered an autoimmune disease. Scientists suspect that certain genes, and perhaps a combination of different genes, predispose people to develop lupus. Genes alone do not determine who will get lupus. Even in genetically susceptible people, some environmental factor, such as an infection, may trigger the disease. Female hormones are believed to play a significant role in lupus.

A major boost to the understanding and treatment of lupus occurred in 2000, with the formation of the Alliance for Lupus Research, a nonprofit partnership between the Arthritis Foundation and New York Jets owner Robert Wood Johnson IV. The Alliance is committed to raising funds that will provide sizable research grants. These grants will go to accomplished researchers whose work is deemed to have the greatest potential to find a cure for SLE within 10 years.

For information about ALR, call 800/867-1743, or visit their web site at www.lupusresearch.org.

BACK PAIN

At some point in their lives, an estimated two-thirds of adults will experience some type of low back pain. The cause may be a day of strenuous activity, an injury suffered in an automobile accident, or a single episode of bending improperly to lift a heavy load.

For some, however, the low back pain is caused by arthritis of the spine. The most common cause of chronic back pain is osteoarthritis. Other arthritis-related causes of back pain include nerves that are compressed or pinched due to bony overgrowth of the spine; fracture or compression of the vertebrae (the bones that make up the spine) due to osteoporosis; and slipped or ruptured disks (the wedges of cartilage that provide cushion between the vertebrae).

Research examining the causes of back pain, who is likely to have it, and why it persists in some people and not others, offers hope for easing or even preventing this common problem. For many people, back pain goes away on its own, with time, regardless of treatment. For

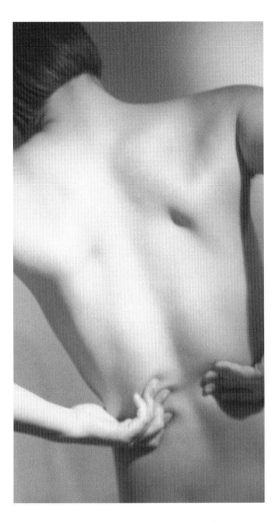

junction with other major forms of arthritis, such as rheumatoid arthritis or lupus. These diseases include the following:

Osteoporosis

The most common disorder of the bone, osteoporosis (or porous bones) is a condition in which the body loses so much bone mass that bones are susceptible to disabling fractures after the slightest trauma. The disease is most common in older women, whose bodies no longer produce large levels of the bone-preserving hormone estrogen.

Some medications used to treat inflammatory forms of arthritis, including such glucocorticoids as prednisone, can increase the risk of developing osteoporosis.

Osteoporosis is not painful. In fact, it's likely that you might never experience symptoms until you suffer a broken bone. Fortunately, the condition can be treated to minimize fracture risk. (See Nutrition for Healthy Bones, page 71.)

Polymyositis

Polymyositis, an inflammation of many muscles, is a disease of generalized weakness that results from inflammation of the muscles, primarily those of the shoulders, upper arms, thighs and hips. Weakness may develop gradually, over the course of months or years, or it can happen suddenly. In some people, polymyositis affects the muscles in the throat or chest, leading to difficulties with swallowing or breathing.

When polymyositis is accompanied by a patchy rash, typically seen over the eyelids, upper chest, neck or hands, doctors refer to the disease as *dermatomyositis*.

others, back pain requires treatment that is targeted to the problem causing the pain.

OTHER RELATED DISEASES

The conditions we have just described are some of the more common diseases that fall into the category of arthritis and related conditions. But there are many other conditions related to arthritis. Some of these conditions may occur in con-

Like many arthritis-related diseases, polymyositis is more common in women than in men, and its development is linked to genetic and environmental factors. Polymyositis occurs most often between the ages of 30 and 60.

Scleroderma

Translated literally as "hard skin," scleroderma results from an abnormal overgrowth of collagen within the skin, in a process called fibrosis. In some forms of the disease, the effects of this abnormal overgrowth are limited to the skin and underlying tissues. In others, however, connective-tissue buildup can affect the function of the joints, blood vessels and internal organs, such as the heart, lungs, kidneys and intestines.

Polymyalgia Rheumatica

Although this term means pain in many muscles, polymyalgia rheumatica (PMR) actually is a disease of the joints. Inflammation in the joints of neck, shoulder and hip areas causes stiffness and aching in those areas. PMR affects an estimated 450,000 people, and approximately 66 percent of them are women. The disease rarely occurs in people before age 50; the average age at which PMR begins is 70.

Sjögren's Syndrome

A condition that affects approximately one million people, 90 percent of whom are women, Sjögren's syndrome is an autoimmune disease that may occur on its own or in conjunction with another disease, such as rheumatoid arthritis, lupus or scleroderma. In people with Sjögren's syndrome, a type of white blood cell called a lymphocyte invades moisture-producing glands, causing inflammation and such problems as dry mouth and eyes.

In addition to tissue dryness, Sjögren's syndrome can cause inflammation in the joints, lungs, kidneys, nerves, thyroid gland and skin.

Infectious Arthritis

As the name implies, infectious arthritis is caused by infection, typically by a bacterium, such as staphylococcus (staph), or a virus, such as hepatitis C. Less commonly, the infection results from a fungus, such as blastomycosis or Candida.

Signs of infectious arthritis differ by the severity of the condition and the type of infection involved. Bacterial infections, for example, most often affect a single joint, typically a large joint, such as the knee. Symptoms of bacterial arthritis include moderate to severe joint pain, swelling, redness and warmth. Such symptoms often come on quickly and may be accompanied by fever and chills. The symptoms of viral-related arthritis depend largely on the particular virus involved. Most types of viral-related arthritis develop gradually and cause widespread joint aches, rather than arthritis in one or a few joints. Fungal infections usually are insidious, with only mild inflammation, but occasionally, fungal infection can cause an acute arthritis in a single joint.

Infectious arthritis can occur in people of any age, but about half of the cases affect people over age 60. Risk factors include having a coexisting disease, such as RA, another inflammatory form of arthritis, diabetes mellitus, chronic liver disease or any condition in which the immune system is suppressed.

Psoriatic Arthritis

As the name suggests, psoriatic arthritis is a form of joint disease accompanied by psoriasis, a disease of the skin that is characterized by thickened, inflamed patches of skin covered by silver-gray scales.

In the majority of people with psoriatic arthritis, the skin disease precedes arthritis by several months or even years. In rare cases, arthritis precedes the skin disease. Psoriatic arthritis affects men and women in equal numbers and generally begins in people between the ages of 30 and 50. In addition to the joints and skin, psoriatic arthritis may affect the nails, causing thickening, pitting and separation from the nail bed.

Osteonecrosis

Also referred to as avascular necrosis, osteonecrosis (literally "bone death") typically affects a segment of the bone and cartilage of the joint, leading to pain and, eventually, loss of movement of the joint. The condition is most common in people between the ages of 30 and 60 and can occur as a complication of glucocorticoid therapy for arthritis or for an injury to the joint.

The most common sites of osteonecrosis are the hip and the knee, but it can develop in any joint. Severe damage to the joint may require a total joint replacement.

Raynaud's Phenomenon

Raynaud's phenomenon is a condition in which the small blood vessels of the hands and feet contract and go into spasms in response to cold or stress. As the vessels contract, the hands or feet turn white and cold, and then blue. As the vessels open and blood flow returns, the hands and feet become red. In severe cases, the tissues in the tips of the fingers and toes may be damaged. Sometimes, Raynaud's phenomenon is associated with an underlying autoimmune disease, such as lupus or scleroderma. It commonly occurs in the absence of arthritis.

Carpal Tunnel Syndrome

Carpal tunnel syndrome occurs when the median nerve, which supplies the thumb side of the hand with sensation, becomes compressed within the wrist. The resulting symptoms can include tingling, numbness and pain in the thumb and the first and middle fingers; shooting pain from the hand, along the arm, to the shoulder; and a swollen feeling in the fingers.

The carpal tunnel, an opening in the bones of the wrist through which the median nerve runs, is narrow, and any swelling or inflammation of the connective tissue that holds together the bones of the wrist can cause pressure on the nerve or irritate it. Causes of inflammation can include injuries to the wrist or forearm, arthritis and activities that require repetitive finger or wrist motion.

Spinal Stenosis

Literally meaning spinal narrowing, spinal stenosis is a condition that occurs when bony overgrowths in the spinal column cause the column to narrow and press on the nerves housed within. Because these nerves have many functions, the condition may cause diverse problems in the lower body, including low back pain, pain or numbness in the legs, constipation and urinary incontinence.

Vasculitis

Vasculitis is an inflammation of the blood vessels that can occur with rheumatoid arthritis and some other inflammatory forms of arthritis. The are many types of vasculitis. The location and effects of vasculitis depend largely on which vessels are affected. In RA, for example, the vessels affected often are those that supply the skin and supporting nerves. The result may be skin ulceration.

In a condition called temporal arteritis, the vessel affected is the artery that supplies the head and scalp. If untreated, temporal arteritis can lead to vision problems and even permanent loss of vision.

UNDERSTANDING WHICH FORM OF ARTHRITIS YOU HAVE

As evident from their descriptions, many forms of arthritis and related conditions share common symptoms. Other diseases also may share the similar symptoms of arthritis, making it impossible to determine on your own which condition you have. Gauging the disease's severity also can be difficult. Some people with severe arthritis report relatively mild pain, while others who have relatively mild arthritis report having severe pain.

Because the specific condition and its severity largely will dictate the treatment you need, it's important to see a doctor for a diagnosis. The following chapter looks at some of the signs that indicate it is time to see a doctor about your joint pain, and it discusses methods your doctor may use to determine which form of arthritis or related condition you have.

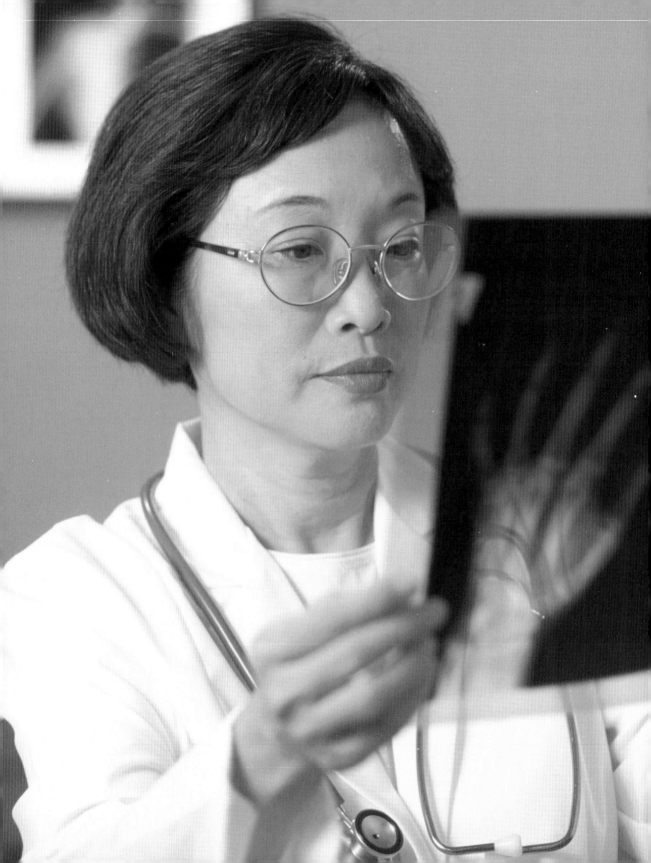

Diagnosing
Arthritis

3

CHAPTER 3: DIAGNOSING ARTHRITIS

Joint and muscle pain can have many causes, some of which are not serious and will resolve with or without treatment. At other times, arthritis can signal a serious problem that requires prompt medical attention to keep it from getting worse. Obviously, it's important to know the difference!

In general, you should consult your doctor if you experience arthritis symptoms that come on suddenly, such as a joint rapidly becoming hot, swollen or difficult to move, or if you have any of the following signs for longer than two weeks:

- Pain in a joint that doesn't go away or keeps returning
- Joint stiffness
- Swelling in a joint, especially with warmth and redness
- Joint or muscle pain accompanied by fatigue, malaise or fever

The first step of a medical evaluation for arthritis probably will be to see your primary-care physician. If your primary doctor doesn't feel confident in diagnosing or treating your condition, or if you or your physician suspect a condition that requires specialized knowledge and care, you should see a rheumatologist. A rheumatologist is a doctor who typically spends three years beyond medical school in an internal medicine residency and at least an additional two to three years specializing in the diagnosis and treatment of arthritis.

Regardless of what kind of doctor you see, the initial evaluation probably will include a physical exam and a medical history.

THE EXAM AND THE MEDICAL HISTORY

The physical exam will vary depending on the type of symptoms you have. Your physician may visually examine, feel and move your joints, and examine your skin, mouth and eyes to check for evidence of a particular form of arthritis.

You probably will be asked to walk, raise your arms and bend over, so the physician can observe your gait and flexibility. He or she may apply pressure to certain points on your body (including points at the base of the skull and around the shoulders, thighs and inner knees) called tender points, which are painful in people with fibromyalgia. (See "The Fibromyalgia Exam" page 35.)

During a medical history, your doctor will ask you about any symptoms, past injuries or illnesses and lifestyle habits, such as smoking, that may be associated with arthritis. Because certain forms of arthritis appear to have a genetic basis, you can expect questions about family members' illnesses, particularly autoimmune and musculoskeletal problems. It's best to become familiar with your family history, if possible, and make notes about any concerns you have before you see the doctor. (For some idea of the type of information you should bring to your first appointment, see, "What to Tell Your Doctor," on the next page.)

In many cases, a doctor who is knowledgeable about the various forms of arthritis and their signs and symptoms can get a pretty good idea of the type of arthritis you have from the exam and medical history.

What To Tell Your Doctor

Thinking about your concerns and writing them down to bring with you when you see your doctor is a handy way to make sure that everything important is discussed. Think about these points before your appointment:

- When the pain started
- What the pain feels like
- How long the pain lasts
- What time of day the pain is worst
- Other symptoms you've noticed
- Other medical conditions you have
- Childhood illnesses you've had
- Adult illnesses you've had
- Surgeries you've had
- Injuries you've had
- Lifestyle habits (bad and good)
- Medical conditions your family members have had

In some cases, your doctor will order or perform medical tests that may provide clues to what's going on in your body and help make a diagnosis or to confirm what they already suspect. The following types of tests may be used to help make or confirm a diagnosis:

Lab Tests

Most lab tests require no more than drawing a small amount of blood or providing a urine sample, but can provide valuable clues to what's occurring elsewhere in the body. Here are some of the most common lab tests.

Erythrocyte Sedimentation Rate. Also referred to as ESR or "sed rate," this blood test measures how fast red blood cells fall to the bottom of a test tube. Because inflammatory substances in the blood make red blood cells cling together and because the clumps that form are heavier and fall faster than single cells, a high sed rate can signal inflammation. The higher the sed rate, the greater the inflammation. Most inflammatory diseases, including rheumatoid arthritis, ankylosing spondylitis, vasculitis, juvenile arthritis and polymyalgia rheumatica, are characterized by a high sed rate.

C-reactive Protein. C-reactive protein appears in the blood during inflammatory processes and thus may be useful in determining if you have an inflammatory form of arthritis. Some doctors use the C-reactive protein test instead of or in conjunction with the erythrocyte sedimentation rate (ESR or sed rate) to monitor the progress of arthritis.

Complete Blood Count (CBC). The CBC is made up of measurements of specific blood components, which can help your doctor diagnose disease and monitor the effects of disease and its treatment. Findings of a CBC might include anemia, which would indicate chronic inflammation, blood loss or perhaps the presence of inflammatory bowel disease; low white blood cell count, which might indicate lupus; high white-blood cell count, which could indicate infection or systemic JRA; or low blood platelets, which could indicate lupus.

Uric Acid. Abnormally high levels of the bodily waste product uric acid in the blood may indicate gout, a condition in which excess uric acid is deposited as crystals in the joints and other tissues (see Chapter 2). To confirm a diagnosis of gout, however, your doctor will need to examine the joint fluid for uric acid crystals.

Urinalysis. Urinalysis refers to a battery of tests used to screen for urinary tract infections, kidney disease and other health problems that can cause changes in the urine. In people with lupus, urinalysis may be used to check for protein and red blood cells, which can indicate kidney inflammation, a condition referred to as lupus nephritis.

Rheumatoid Factor (RF) Test (or RA latex test). The presence of rheumatoid factor (RF), an autoantibody that is produced in large amounts in people with rheumatoid arthritis, can help a doctor diagnose that disease. Approximately 80 percent of people with RA test positive for rheumatoid factor. However, because a smaller percentage of people without RA also test positive, the presence of RF in the blood doesn't confirm a diagnosis.

Antinuclear Antibody (ANA). Antinuclear antibodies are antibodies directed against the nuclei, or command centers, of the body's cells. ANAs can be found in approximately 95 percent of people with lupus. These antibodies also can be found in many other forms of arthritis, including rheumatoid arthritis, scleroderma, polymyositis and Sjögren's syndrome, and they sometimes are found in low amounts (called 'low titers') in healthy people. Used in conjunction with other tests, ANA can help diagnose these diseases.

Anti-DNA. Antibodies to DNA (deoxyribonucleic acid, the hereditary material in the nucleus of every cell) are common in people with lupus. Because these antibodies rarely are found in people with any other disease, the finding of anti-DNA antibodies in the blood is used to diagnose lupus.

Complement. When antibodies combine with invading agents, a substance in the blood called *complement* aids the body's immune defenses. Blood samples showing low levels of complement can suggest such inflammatory conditions as lupus or vasculitis. Other tests are necessary, however, to aid in the diagnosis of these diseases.

Joint Fluid Exam. The examination of fluid withdrawn from the joint cavity can help your doctor diagnose gout or infectious arthritis. In gout, crystals of uric acid – a bodily waste product – can be found in the joint fluid. The finding of bacteria in the joint fluid indicates infectious arthritis.

Lyme Serology. To confirm a diagnosis of Lyme disease, blood is tested for antibodies that are made in response to Borrelia Burgdorferi, the spirochete (spiral-shaped bacterium) that causes the disease.

Tissue Typing. The finding of a specific genetic marker called HLA-B27 in the blood through tissue typing helps confirm a diagnosis of ankylosing spondylitis, a form of arthritis that primarily affects the spine and sacroiliac joints, or reactive arthritis, a similar disease that is char-

acterized by inflammation of the joints, eyes and urethra. The finding of a marker called HLA-DR4 may indicate RA.

Imaging Tests

Imaging studies are used to view components of the body to detect and assess signs of arthritis. Your doctor may order one of the following radiologic tests.

X-rays. Plain X-rays often are used in the diagnosis of arthritis because they enable a physician to view the bony structures that make up the joint. X-rays can show such problems as fluid accumulation in the joint, cartilage damage, patterns of cartilage wear and abnormalities of bone. These signs can help doctors determine which form of arthritis you have.

In osteoarthritis, the joint space (the area between the two bones that make up the joint) may appear narrow and uneven because of the irregular wear and damage that OA causes to the cartilage. The ends of the bones may appear dense, and there may be evidence of bony growths called spurs. Rheumatoid arthritis, on the other hand, causes more consistent joint-space narrowing. X-rays may show bone thinning around the joint or bone erosion.

X-rays also show certain bony changes in the spine, which helps doctors diagnose ankylosing spondylitis and other spondyloarthropathies. Other forms of arthritis, such as psoriatic arthritis, also show characteristic patterns of joint damage on X-rays, enabling doctors to differentiate them.

Sometimes a doctor will inject dye into a joint before X-raying it, a procedure called arthrography. The dye helps illuminate the spaces inside the joints and enables your doctor to view and diagnose such problems as damage to the cartilage, supporting muscles, tendons and ligaments.

DEXA scans. Dual energy X-ray absorptiometry (DEXA) scans are the most reliable way to diagnose osteoporosis and determine a person's risk for a bone fracture.

A DEXA scan is similar to an X-ray, except that it uses much less radiation. Having a DEXA scan involves lying on a table while an imaging machine passes over you, measuring bone density at the hip and spine. The procedure is painless and usually takes 15 to 20 minutes.

Because osteoporosis is such a common and potentially dangerous problem for women who are past menopause, some doctors recommend a routine DEXA scan for all women five to 10 years after menopause. If you have an inflammatory disease, such as RA or lupus, your doctor may order a DEXA scan regardless of your age, particularly if you take a glucocorticoid medication for the disease.

MRI. Magnetic resonance imaging (MRI) is a procedure in which a very strong magnet passes a force through the body to create a clear, detailed image of a cross-section of the body. The procedure is harmless and does not expose the body to radiation.

The advantage of MRI scans over plain X-rays is that MRI provides detailed images of such soft-tissue structures as the synovium, tendons, ligaments and muscles, as well as bone.

Arthritis-related uses for MRI include diagnosing avascular necrosis of the hip; ankylosing spondylitis, spinal stenosis and other back-related problems; injuries to the soft tissues of the knee; and less commonly, other types of joint problems.

Having an MRI typically involves lying on a long, narrow table that slides into a large, tunnel-like tube within the scanner. Several images are taken of the joint or organ being examined. Each image takes between two and 15 minutes; the entire procedure takes about an hour.

In the past, people who were claustrophobic were not good candidates for MRI because the procedure requires being confined in a small space. In recent years, however, a type of machine called open MRI has been introduced that is less confining than traditional models. Although the images these newer machines produce may not be of the same quality as those produced by traditional machines, they do make MRI an option for more people.

If you wear a pacemaker or have any type of metal implant in your body (including implants for orthopaedic reasons) either type of MRI may be inappropriate for you. If you have concerns about MRI, it's best to discuss them with your doctor beforehand.

Ultrasonography. Increasingly, doctors are using ultrasonography – the use of sound waves to produce pictures of structures within the body – in the diagnosis of arthritis and related diseases. Benefits of ultrasonography, often referred to as ultrasound, are that it doesn't use radiation and it can take pictures of the body's soft tissues.

Ultrasound can be useful in the diagnosis of such problems as bursitis, an inflammation of the bursae that cushion the shoulder, and plantar fasciitis, a tear in a ligament in the arch of the foot. Doctors also use ultrasonography to assess inflammation of the synovium, the membrane that lines the joint, and to detect the presence of fluid within the joint cavity.

Biopsies

Biopsies are tests performed on pieces of bodily tissue that are removed surgically, most often through small incisions. Depending on the piece of tissue examined, your doctor may use a biopsy to diagnose diseases of the joint, muscle, skin or blood vessels. Following are descriptions of biopsies often used to diagnose arthritis and related diseases.

Muscle. Used in the diagnosis of polymyositis or dermatomyositis, a muscle biopsy involves removing a sample of muscle, usually from the thigh, through a small incision.

Skin. Used to diagnose or confirm a diagnosis of lupus or vasculitis, a skin biopsy is obtained with a special needle inserted into the skin. The tissue usually is taken from an area where a small scar would not be very noticeable.

Synovium. Biopsy of the synovium (the joint lining) can help diagnose various forms of arthritis. To remove a sample of the synovium, your doctor will insert a special biopsy needle into the joint. A synovial biopsy also can be obtained by a procedure called arthroscopy, which is discussed later in this section.

Temporal artery. Temporal artery biopsy is performed to help diagnose giant cell arteritis (GCA), also called temporal arteritis. The procedure involves making an inch-long vertical incision in front of the ear and removing a small segment of the temporal artery for examination.

Kidney biopsy. Kidney biopsy involves inserting a special needle through an incision in the lower back and removing a small sample of kidney for examination. If you have lupus, and urinalysis shows evidence of kidney inflammation, a kidney biopsy can be used to confirm a diagnosis of lupus nephritis.

Arthroscopy

Doctors sometimes use a surgical procedure called arthroscopy to diagnose or evaluate joint problems. In arthroscopy, a thin tube with a light at the end, called an arthroscope, is inserted directly into the joint through a small incision. The arthroscope, which is attached to a closed-circuit television, illuminates the interior of the joint and enables your doctor to see it on the screen.

The procedure typically is performed under local or spinal anesthesia on an outpatient basis. If a problem is detected through arthroscopy, the damage often can be repaired during the same procedure.

Although the use of arthroscopy is far from routine in the diagnosis of arthritis-related problems, it commonly is used to remove loose pieces of tissue that cause pain, repair torn cartilage, or smooth rough joint surfaces. Arthroscopy sometimes is used for more extensive surgery, such as ligament reconstruction and *synovectomy*, the removal of a diseased joint lining. For more information about arthroscopy, see Chapter 8.

Diagnosis Difficulties

Some arthritis-related diseases are fairly rare. A doctor who doesn't specialize in arthritis treatment, such as a primary-care physician, may never have seen a patient with that particular disease and may have difficulty diagnosing it. Even for a specialized doctor, arriving at a precise diagnosis can take time. Here, we will look at some of the reasons why this occurs.

- **Same symptoms, different diseases.** Some forms of arthritis share characteristics with one another or with unrelated diseases. For example, joint pain and inflammation can be a symptom of many diseases. Without diagnostic tests, it may be difficult for a clinician to differentiate between RA and ankylosing spondylitis or between RA and gout. Raynaud's phenomenon, a condition in which the fingers blanch in response to cold temperatures or emotional stress (see chapter 2), can be an early symptom of both lupus and scleroderma.

- **Same person, different diseases.** Because a person can have more than one form of arthri-

tis simultaneously, sorting through which condition is causing what problem may take some time. For example, a person with lupus may have hip pain that is caused by osteonecrosis. A person with RA may have a swollen knee due to infectious arthritis.

- **Disease evolution.** Some forms of arthritis can take months or years to completely reveal themselves. Blood tests that once were negative may, when repeated, become positive. A pattern of joint involvement or other symptoms may become more pronounced or clearer. Some forms of arthritis that accompany viral infections can mimic RA or other conditions, but resolve on their own, usually after a few weeks.

The diagnosis process may not occur quickly or exactly as you would hope or expect. In most cases, however, your doctor can give you a pretty good idea of what's going on, even if a precise diagnosis takes some time.

Treatment likely will depend on the particular form of arthritis or related condition you have, but a precise diagnosis often is not essential before beginning treatment. What's most important early on is that you are being seen by a doctor who can help minimize the symptoms of your condition. Perhaps, your doctor will give you a medication that will keep your condition from worsening or causing irreparable joint or organ damage.

THE FIBROMYALGIA EXAM

For many forms of arthritis and related conditions, positive results on certain lab tests can help a doctor make or confirm a diagnosis. For fibromyalgia, however, there are no routine lab tests to confirm or rule out the condition. In diagnosing fibromyalgia, the history and physical exam take on added importance.

One of the key determinants of a fibromyalgia diagnosis is the presence of tender points, which are tender, painful areas in the muscles, tendons or other areas of the body where the bone can be felt through the skin. Many people with fibromyalgia don't even realize they have tender points until the physician applies pressure to them.

The location of these tender points is fairly consistent from person to person. There are 18 recognized tender points in fibromyalgia. In general, to be diagnosed with fibromyalgia, you must have at least 11 of these tender points in combination with widespread pain.

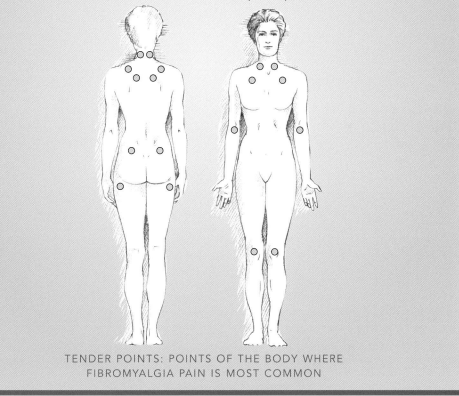

TENDER POINTS: POINTS OF THE BODY WHERE
FIBROMYALGIA PAIN IS MOST COMMON

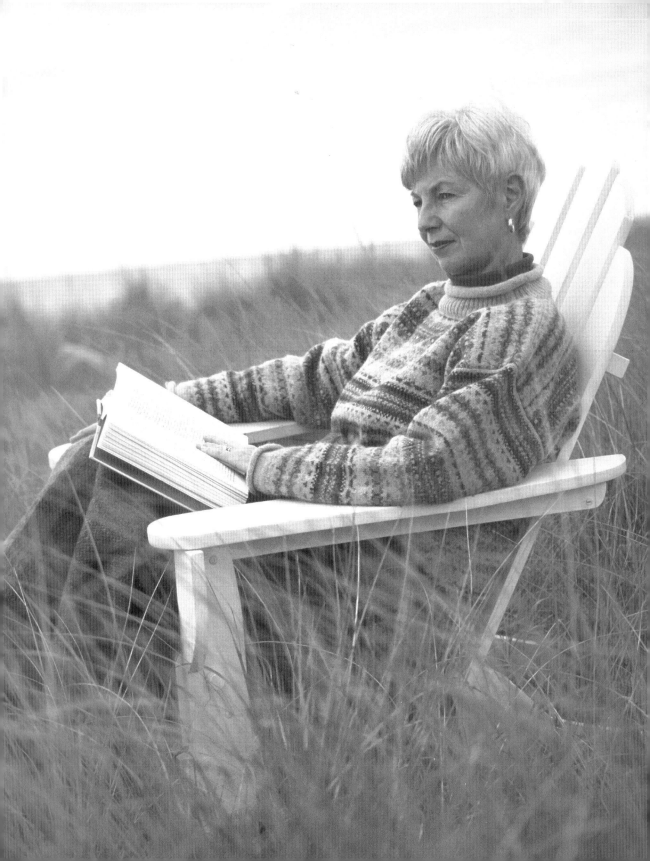

After the Diagnosis

4

CHAPTER 4: AFTER THE DIAGNOSIS

Getting a diagnosis can bring mixed emotions. It can be upsetting and frightening to learn that you have a chronic disease – that your problem may be more serious than "aches and pains." However, you may feel a sense of relief to have a name for what has been troubling you. Regardless of the way your diagnosis affects you emotionally, try to remember that a diagnosis is a positive step. It allows you to learn more about your specific medical condition and what you and your doctor can do to help you get better.

GETTING PROPER CARE – A TEAM EFFORT

If you have been seeing a primary-care physician up to the point of your diagnosis, you may be referred to or may choose to see a rheumatologist or orthopaedic surgeon, depending on the diagnosis. Rheumatologists are doctors who specialize in treating arthritis and related conditions. Orthopaedic surgeons treat diseases of the bone and joints.

Although most cases of osteoarthritis may be treated quite effectively by a general internist or family physician, diseases such as lupus and RA may require the knowledge and experience of a specialist.

If you feel you need to see a rheumatologist, your primary-care physician can recommend one, although in some cases, your health insurance may dictate the rheumatologist you will see. Another way to find a reputable rheumatologist is by contacting your local Arthritis

Foundation chapter for a list of doctors in your area. You can locate your chapter by calling 800/283-7800 or by visiting www.arthritis.org. You can ask family, friends or coworkers for recommendations, or check the Web site of the American College of Rheumatology, (www.rheumatology.org), or the American Academy of Orthopaedic Surgeons (www.aaos.org) which maintains a listing of specialists by state.

Members of Your Health-Care Team

At some point, you may seek the services of other health-care professionals, including specialized physicians, to help you manage the various aspects of your disease. In addition to a rheumatologist or an orthopaedist, the people who may be part of your health-care team include the following professionals:

Other doctors. Because different forms of arthritis can be systemic, meaning that they affect the entire body, your care may involve seeing doctors who specialize in treating organs and systems affected by arthritis-related disease. In addition to rheumatologists and orthopaedic surgeons, these doctors may include dermatologists, who specialize in treating problems of the skin, hair and nails; ophthalmologists, who specialize in problems of the eyes; nephrologists, who specialize in kidney disease; geriatricians, who specialize in the treatment of older people; and pediatric rheumatologists, who specialize in treating arthritis in children.

WORKING WITH YOUR DOCTOR: FINDING THE RIGHT FIT

Managing your arthritis requires a team effort. But what if your doctor doesn't want to be a part of the team? Many doctors appreciate informed, involved patients, but there are exceptions.

Some doctors view a patient's questions as a sign of distrust or are put off by patients who want to take charge of their own health care. For some patients, such doctors are fine. Just as there are doctors who want you to follow their orders – period – there are patients who prefer to put all of their medical decisions in the hands of the physician. These patients find comfort in knowing that someone else is in charge.

While the best doctor-patient relationship is one in which there is some give-and-take, what's most important is that you see eye-to-eye with your doctor. Problems arise when there is a discrepancy between the way you and your doctor prefer to work. If you want to take a role in your health care, but your doctor expects you to follow orders without question, it may be time to find a new doctor.

Before you switch, however, be sure that you're not asking for or expecting too much. Although your doctor should be willing to answer questions and be open to the possibility of different treatments you would like to try, no doctor has the time to answer endless lists of queries from every patient.

A doctor who merely agrees with everything you suggest is not good for you. And prescribing or condoning every treatment you mention can be downright dangerous.

Doctors can be either MDs (medical doctors) or DOs (doctors of osteopathic medicine). Other than some differences in philosophy, MDs and DOs have similar training and skills, and both can prescribe medication and provide appropriate medical care.

Physician assistant. Physician assistants are health-care professionals licensed to practice medicine with a physician's supervision, and they may practice in primary and specialty care in medical and surgical practice settings. Physician assistants can give injections, perform some diagnostic tests and discuss your disease and treatment plan.

Physical therapist. If arthritis causes pain and limited motion in your joints, or causes difficulties with walking, stretching, bending or climbing stairs, a physical therapist (PT) may help. A PT can devise an exercise plan that strengthens your muscles and increases your range of motion. PTs also prescribe such devices as canes, splints or shoe inserts. Many PTs are trained in soft-tissue massage, which people with arthritis often find helpful to relieve pain and stiffness.

Occupational therapist. An occupational therapist (OT) can help you find ways to manage daily tasks at home and on the job. If arthritis makes it difficult to handle such tasks as cooking, typing, driving, brushing your teeth or buttoning your clothes, an OT may suggest different ways to do these tasks or prescribe assistive devices or splints. Some OTs earn the designation of certified hand therapist (CHT), by completing specialized training to help patients with problems related to the elbows, hands and wrists.

Registered nurse. In addition to taking your blood pressure, drawing blood and providing routine care, nurses function as patient educators and advocates. When you call the doctor's office for help, a nurse often will be the one to return your call, and you may spend more time talking with the nurses in your doctor's office than talking with your doctor. In some cases, you may see a nurse practitioner, which is a nurse with advanced training who is qualified to interpret lab tests and, in most states, prescribe medication.

Registered dietitian. Diet and weight management are important in arthritis, because excess weight can add stress to fragile joints and can complicate joint surgery. A proper diet can help you reduce your risk of other health problems, such as diabetes, cardiovascular disease and some cancers. A consultation with a dietitian may help you find a healthful diet that fits your lifestyle.

Psychologist and social worker. When you're struggling with a chronic disease, it's understandable that you may get depressed. Mental-health professionals can help you deal with the psychological aspects of your illness, such as depression, anxiety and anger. Social workers can help with the practical aspects of disease, such as finding appropriate health insurance and housing.

Psychologists and social workers cannot prescribe medications. If you have a problem that requires or would be helped by medication, they will refer you to a psychiatrist. Psychiatrists are medical doctors with psychiatric training who can prescribe such medications as antidepressants.

Pharmacist. No matter which type of arthritis you have, there is a good chance that you will take some type of medication for it. Your pharmacist can be a good source of information about the medications your doctor prescribes and the medications you purchase over the counter. Don't hesitate to ask your pharmacist questions about side effects, how to take medication or which brands of over-the-counter medications are appropriate for you.

Podiatrist. A podiatrist, or doctor of podiatric medicine (DPM), treats conditions of the foot, from nail infections to arthritis-damaged joints.

Also called foot-and-ankle surgeons, podiatrists are licensed to perform surgery and prescribe medications. If arthritis affects your feet, you may choose a podiatrist to be a member of your health-care team.

Dentist. If Sjögren's syndrome causes dry mouth, if arthritis affects your jaw joint (a condition called temporomandibular joint disorder) or makes it difficult to perform proper oral hygiene, you're particularly vulnerable to dental problems. For that reason, it's especially imp-

ortant that you see a dentist regularly to detect and take care of any problems before they become severe. In addition, a dentist may offer advice on how to brush and floss your teeth if arthritis affects your hands.

Acupuncturist. If you need help with pain and are willing to try an alternative therapy, you may want to see an acupuncturist. Acupuncturists insert slender needles into the skin at various points on the body to relieve pain. The theory behind acupuncture is that the practice corrects

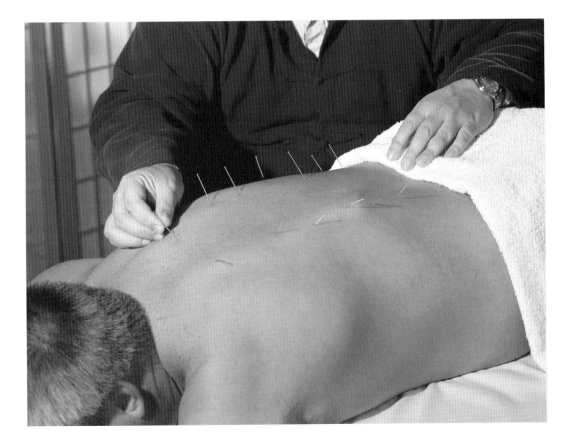

the flow of *qi*, the body's vital energy, which optimizes health. Modern research suggests that acupuncture may ease pain by causing the release of endorphins. Although most acupuncturists are not physicians, some of them are. Check an acupuncturist's credentials before you make your appointment.

Massage therapist. You know how good it feels to have your back and shoulders rubbed when you are achy and stiff. Massage therapists are specially trained and certified to perform therapeutic massage, which can relieve muscle tension, improve range of motion and, perhaps, ease pain.

Chiropractor. Formally referred to as doctors of chiropractic medicine (DC), chiropractors use manual manipulation of the joints to increase range of motion and help relieve pain.

For people with certain types of arthritis, however, manipulations may not be indicated or safe. Chiropractors do not perform surgery or prescribe medication.

The health-care professionals you see and the treatment you receive will depend on a number of factors, including the type of arthritis you have, your symptoms and their severity, your insurance coverage, treatment preferences of you and your doctor, and your general physical condition, including any other medical problems you have and medications you take for them.

Regardless of which or how many people are on your team, it's important that you have an honest give-and-take relationship with the person, usually your rheumatologist or primary-care physician, who coordinates your arthritis care.

Your doctor probably will discuss lifestyle issues in addition to your medical treatment. Are you physically active or sedentary most of the time? Are you trim or overweight? Do you eat a varied diet, with plenty of fruits and vegetables? Do you smoke? All of these factors can influence your general health and your arthritis. If your doctor doesn't bring up these issues, you should. Although medication and other treatments are important in arthritis, a big part of your treatment's success has to do with you. *You* should be the leader of your health-care team.

THE IMPORTANCE OF INFORMATION – AND WHERE TO FIND IT

As the leader of your health-care team, you need to arm yourself with knowledge. Being informed enables you to talk more confidently with your doctor and other health-care professionals. It also can help you understand which symptoms need to be brought to your doctor's attention immediately and which symptoms should resolve without treatment. Being knowledgeable also makes you aware of potential treatments you can discuss with your doctors and gives you a sense of control that has been shown repeatedly in studies to improve the outcome of disease.

Although you will get much of your information from the doctor, your quest for knowledge should not stop at the doctor's office. Today, more than ever, information is available to help you understand and manage your disease – if you know where to look.

MEDICAL RESEARCH: SEPARATE FACT FROM FICTION

Today, more than ever, consumers have access to an abundance of information about arthritis and other topics. Although much of what you read may be accurate and helpful, a great deal of the information you'll find in publications and on the Internet is not. Even good, accurate information may not apply to your particular situation or your form of arthritis.

How can you separate the good from the bad, useless or dangerous? Evaluate everything you read with the following criteria:

Consider the source. Was it published in a peer-reviewed journal? The most reliable studies are those published in reputable journals, which have been reviewed by other doctors before publication. Vague references to being scientifically tested may mean nothing.

Who did the research? Was the research conducted by an institution that is familiar to you? Does the article say who funded the study? A study conducted at a major medical center may be more reputable than one conducted by a single physician in his private practice, although there are exceptions. Research funded by the Arthritis Foundation or the National Institutes of Health, for example, is more likely to be reliable than research funded by the manufacturer of an unfamiliar arthritis remedy. However, pharmaceutical companies sponsor much of the research into treatments for arthritis, and they play an important role in bringing new drugs to the marketplace. Your doctor should be in a good position to evaluate the credibility of a study.

Who was studied? Although the research may be solid, it may mean nothing for you if the people in the study were in a different situation from yours. In other words, a new drug that looks promising in 100 women with rheumatoid arthritis may be of no use for a man with osteoarthritis.

Have you seen similar reports elsewhere? When evaluating a report in a magazine or newspaper or on a Web site, check around to see if you can find similar information elsewhere. When writing about technical medical topics, it's easy for a writer to get facts wrong. If you see consistent reports in several locations, however, the information is likely to be correct.

Is the article trying to sell you something? Be wary of articles written to promote a product or articles that use sensational claims and anecdotes rather than verifiable, scientific information.

One of your first stops for information should be the Arthritis Foundation. Through its publications (books, brochures, newsletters and *Arthritis Today* magazine) and Web site, the Foundation offers a wealth of information on many arthritis-related subjects – and much of it is free. The Foundation also offers courses where you can learn more about your particular disease and meet and talk to others who are managing problems similar to yours.

To find an Arthritis Foundation office in your area, call 800/283-7800 or visit the Arthritis Foundation's Web site at www.arthritis.org. Let's look at other potential sources of arthritis information on the following pages.

Your Health-Care Provider

In addition to your local Arthritis Foundation office, your doctor, nurse, pharmacist and other health-care professionals may have handouts or brochures on your condition. They also may be able to direct you to helpful classes, support groups or seminars, or even to another patient with your same condition who can offer first-hand advice and lend moral support.

Your Local Library

Most local libraries have a collection of medical reference books, such as medical dictionaries or encyclopedias, medical and nursing handbooks, directories of physicians, and books on drug information. While reference books such as these usually are not available for checkout, you can use them to look up information and make photocopies of pertinent pages for a nominal fee.

Your local library probably has collection of consumer magazines, either in hard copy or on microfilm, containing information on a variety of health topics. Articles run the gamut, from the warning signs and treatments for specific diseases to getting along with your doctor. You can locate magazine articles on particular topics by looking them up in the *Reader's Guide to Periodical Literature.*

If you have access to a medical library, you'll have considerably more resources from which to choose, including computer databases and medical journals and textbooks. Sometimes your community library can get medical books and journals on loan from a larger library if you ask. Keep in mind that most of the information you will find is targeted to physicians. If you have difficulty understanding an article that seems interesting or relevant to you, make a photocopy or make notes to take along on your next visit to your physician, who may be able to help you decipher it.

The Bookstore

Bookstores offer a wealth of information, which may include health magazines, such as *Arthritis Today*, and books written for the consumer. All Arthritis Foundation books are stocked in bookstores nationwide, and if the book is not in stock, it usually can be ordered. If you find a book at the library that is particularly helpful, you can buy a copy at your local bookstore. If you can't find a particular book at your local bookstore, ask them to order it. If you have Internet access, you can get virtually any book, including Arthritis Foundation books, from online booksellers, including www.booksense.com, www.borders.com, www.amazon.com and www.barnesandnoble.com.

You can order any Arthritis Foundation book by calling 800/207-8633, or from the Web site (www.arthritis.org). You also can find Arthritis Foundation books, brochures and other educational materials at your local Arthritis Foundation chapter. Check your telephone directory or call 800/283-7800 to find the chapter nearest you.

Other Voluntary Health Organizations

Depending on your specific arthritis-related problem, you may find helpful information from such organizations as the Scleroderma Foundation, Sjögren's Syndrome Foundation, Lupus Foundation of America or National Osteoporosis Foundation. To locate a local chapter of one of these organizations, check your local phone book or visit their Web sites.

The Federal Government

Another good source of written information about the various arthritis-related diseases is the National Institute of Arthritis and Musculoskeletal and Skin Diseases (NIAMS) Information Clearinghouse. The NIAMS clearinghouse is one of several clearinghouses and information centers operated by the federal government.

To obtain information from the NIAMS clearinghouse, call 301/495-4494 (in Maryland) or 877/22-NIAMS (toll free) or write to:

NIAMS/National Institutes of Health
1 AMS Circle
Bethesda, MD 20892-3675

To obtain a free list of other Federal information clearinghouses, visit the National Health Information Center's home page (www.NHICnt.health.org), write to P.O. Box 1133, Washington, DC 20013-1133, or call 800-336-4707.

Services among these centers vary, but may include publications, referrals and answers to consumer inquiries.

NIAMS also offers a great deal of consumer health information on many forms of arthritis and related diseases on its Web site, www.nih.gov./niams.

The Internet

The Internet is a network of computers throughout the world that can exchange information almost instantaneously. The World Wide Web is a system of electronic documents linked together and available on the Internet to anyone with a computer, a modem and an Internet service provider, such as America Online, CompuServe or EarthLink. Many libraries have Internet access.

If you have access to the Internet, you can find just about any type of information you could want. Some of the sources of information you can find on the Internet include:

- **The Arthritis Foundation.** The Foundation's Web site (www.arthritis.org) is packed with helpful services, including a database of arthritis information searchable by key word; articles from current and past issues of *Arthritis Today*; information about Foundation programs, services and events; locations of Foundation chapters; online ordering of free brochures and other publications; a virtual store, where you can purchase arthritis-friendly products; and message boards that allow you to share tips and experiences and benefit from the input of other people with arthritis. In addition, the site has an interactive self-management page called *Connect and Control*, where you can plug in your personal health information and get advice tailored to your needs.

- **Other voluntary health organizations.** Organizations such as the Lupus Foundation of America (www.lupus.org), National Osteoporosis Foundation (www.nof.org) and Scleroderma Foundation (www.scleroderma.org) have Web sites that offer useful information about specific forms of arthritis.

- **Doctor's organizations.** Every group of medical specialists has a professional society, such as the American College of Rheumatology (www.rheumatology.org), American Academy of Orthopaedic Surgeons (www.aaos.org), American Academy of Dermatology (www.aad.org), American Academy of Family Physicians (www.aafp.org), American College of Physicians (www.acoponline.org), and American Academy of Pediatrics (www.aap.org). Such Web sites may include health information targeted to consumers and links to the organizations' medical journals.

- **Medical journals.** The contents of many medical journals (including those of past issues) can be found on the Internet. While the majority of journals offer full articles only to paid

subscribers, many provide abstracts of articles free of charge to anyone who visits their Web sites. Some sites allow you to purchase the full text of a single study. To locate journals specific to arthritis and related diseases, visit www.mednets.com/rheumatojournals.htm.

- **The National Institute of Arthritis and Musculoskeletal and Skin Diseases (NIAMS).** A branch of the National Institutes of Health, NIAMS offers a variety of publications and other reliable, medically reviewed information on arthritis and related diseases that can be downloaded free of charge. You'll find information about NIAMS at www.nih.gov/niams.

- **The National Library of Medicine.** Operated by the federal government, the library allows you to search its MEDLINE database – one of the largest, best known databases of medical information – free of charge. Once you have located a reference to an articles of interests, you can order copies for a fee. Visit the library's Web site at www.nlm.nih.gov.

- **Universities, pharmaceutical companies and hospitals.** There are countless other sources of arthritis information on the Internet, from university medical centers to commercial Web sites designed to sell products. If you enter the word arthritis in any Internet search engine, you're likely to find thousands of matches. A few examples of good search engines are www. yahoo.com, www.excite. com and www.lycos.com.

- **Message boards and on-line support groups.** Message boards and on-line support groups let you "talk" and share your thoughts, feelings, questions and suggestions with people from around the world. The Arthritis Foundation's Web site contains active message boards that let you chat with other people who have arthritis or related diseases. To read and post messages on the Arthritis Foundation's message board visit the Foundation's Web site (www.arthritis.org) and click on Message Boards in the navigational bar.

In these sources, you will find virtually limitless information that covers a variety of topics, including medications, nutritional supplements and non-medical interventions and treatments.

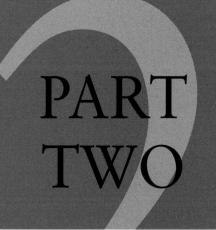

PART TWO

TWO

TREATMENTS FOR ARTHRITIS

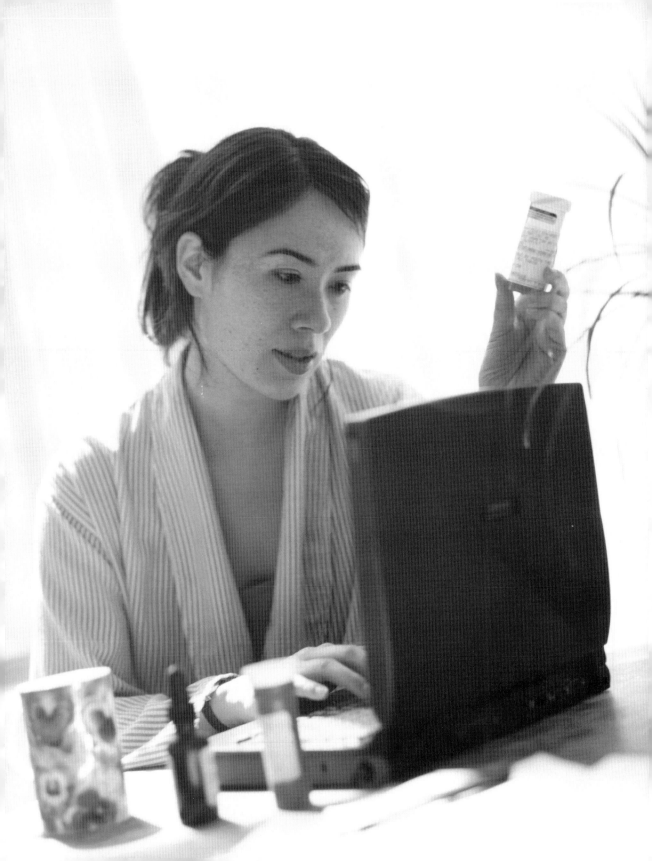

Taking Drugs
For Arthritis

5

CHAPTER 5:
TAKING DRUGS FOR ARTHRITIS

Regardless of the type of arthritis you have or the kind of doctor you see, medications are likely to be part of your arthritis treatment plan. For that reason, it's as important to understand as much as you can about arthritis medications as it is to learn about the medical condition itself.

In Chapter 6, we'll discuss in some detail the various types of medication used to treat the different forms of arthritis and related diseases. However, as you begin to talk to your doctor about medication options or fill your first prescription for arthritis medication, you'll probably have more general questions, which we'll try to answer here.

GENERIC VS. BRAND NAME

When you're filling a prescription, the pharmacist may ask you, "Do you want the generic?" How should you answer? Is a generic as good as the brand-name medication? What's the difference?

As far as you're concerned, the only difference probably is the cost. Choosing generics is likely to cost you significantly less than buying the brand-name counterpart. It is similar to the difference between the store-brand green beans and the brand-name variety. Aside from the product's packaging and, perhaps, minor differences in its appearance, you are getting essentially the same vegetable – or medicine.

Here's why: When a company develops a new drug, it applies for a patent, which prohibits anyone else from marketing the drug for 20 years. This time of exclusivity allows the company to recoup the costs of developing and testing the drug, which averages about $360 million per medication. After the patent has expired, other manufacturers may duplicate and market their own versions of the drug, called generics. Because makers of generic drugs don't have to repeat the extensive clinical trials to prove the safety and efficacy of their drugs, their expenses are much less and they can pass along those savings to you.

Although manufacturers of generic medications don't have to repeat the same rigorous tests that the manufacturer of the original drug must pass (see sidebar on clinical trials), they still must meet certain requirements. They must prove that their drug is chemically identical to the brand-name version (that is, its active ingredient is the same). However, the nonactive ingredients, such as dyes and fillers, may be different. So if you are allergic to certain dyes or fillers, such as corn, that could be an important difference between generic and brand-name medications.

Unfortunately, these nonactive ingredients don't appear on the medications' labels, so the only way you can know how you will react to a generic is to try one. In the vast majority of cases, you'll probably never know the difference. In the rare event that you don't get the same relief as you do from the brand-name medication, or if you experience a reaction to a non-active ingredient in a particular medication, your best bet is to try the same medication from another manufacturer. Ask your doctor or pharmacist for a recommendation.

PRESCRIPTION VS. OVER THE COUNTER

You're scanning the shelves of your local pharmacy for something to ease your aching joints and you find literally dozens of medications labeled as a pain reliever, non-aspirin pain reliever, arthritis formula or nighttime pain reliever. What is the difference between all of these medications, and how do they differ from the medications a doctor prescribes?

Essentially, the difference between these drugs and prescription medications is that you don't need a doctor's written order or phone call to the pharmacy to get them. But they still are serious medicine.

When it comes to arthritis medications, the two types you'll find over the counter are the analgesic medication acetaminophen (*Tylenol*) and four nonsteroidal anti-inflammatory drugs (*NSAIDs*): ibuprofen (*Advil, Motrin*), naproxen sodium (*Aleve*), ketoprofen (*Orudis KT*) and aspirin (*Anacin, Bayer, Bufferin, Excedrin*). Although these drugs come in many formulations and in combination with other ingredients – such as caffeine to speed pain relief, antihistamines to cause drowsiness or a diuretic to ease bloating – these are the only over-the-counter medications you'll find to ease pain.

Increasingly, drugs that were once available only by prescription are becoming available over the counter. Between 1984 and 1994 about one drug per year switched from prescription-only to over-the-counter. In 1996 alone, 13 drugs became available over the counter.

The increasing availability of medications without a doctors' prescription has benefits and drawbacks. On the positive side, getting a medication has never been more convenient and less expensive. You don't need an appointment with a physician just to get a medication or other type of treatment to ease the pain of a muscle strain or a mild ache in your joints.

On the negative side, people are more likely than ever to self-medicate, not realizing they have a condition that requires the care of a physician. People also tend to think that anything they get over the counter is safe and that they can adjust the dosage as they see fit. This belief is not true. Even if you are taking an over-the-counter medication, it's important to follow the directions exactly. You also should contact your doctor promptly if you suspect an adverse reaction or if symptoms don't improve.

It's important to understand that over-the-counter medications may be similar or identical to the ones prescribed by your doctor. Taking an over-the-counter medication along with your prescription may lead to an overdose. Tell your doctor about all the medications you are taking at any time, including over-the-counter treatments.

Fortunately, over-the-counter medications are getting new labels that will help people understand what's in them and how to take them. For more information see, "A Makeover for Medication Labels" on page 106.

Questions to Ask Your Doctor About Drugs

To get the greatest benefit – and least risk of adverse effects – from your medications, it's important to know as much as possible about what your doctor is prescribing. Here are some questions you might want to ask:

- What is the name of the medication?
- What type of drug is this medication?
- How is this medication expected to help me?
- Are there any special instructions for taking this drug?
- Are there side effects?
- What should I do if I experience side effects?
- How long should I expect to wait before noticing effects?
- What should I do if I miss a dose of this medication?
- Is a generic available?
- Will my insurance cover this medication?
- If the medication is too expensive, is there something similar that costs less?
- Is there anything else I should know about this medication?

TRADITIONAL VS. ALTERNATIVE

Before a medication can make it to market, it must first undergo a rigorous process to demonstrate its safety and effectiveness. Based on the results of numerous studies, the Food and Drug Administration (FDA) gives its approval for the drug to be marketed.

Alternative medications, such as the nutritional supplements and herbal remedies you find in health-food stores and in your grocery store's natural remedies section, are not required to undergo that rigorous process, so there is no proof that the alternative remedy will be effective or safe. There also are no assurances that the package will contain what the label says. In fact, some recent studies by an independent lab showed that several products included potentially harmful ingredients that were not listed on the product labels. Many products did not contain the ingredients promised or they contained smaller amounts of ingredients than were listed on the labels.

If you're interested in trying an alternative medication, it's important that you speak with your doctor. Some supplements may interact with over the counter or prescription medications, putting you at risk of dangerous side effects. For more information about alternative medication, see Chapter 12, "Alternative Therapies for Arthritis."

TAKING MEDICATIONS RESPONSIBLY

In most cases, your doctor will decide the medication you need and write the prescription for it, but you are the one who must fill the prescription and take it at the intervals and in the way prescribed. You must report any problems with the medication to your doctor. Remember, you are the leader of your health-care team. When it comes to taking medications, you are in control. With that position of control comes responsibility.

Failure to take medications correctly can cause numerous problems, ranging from failure to obtain the medication's full benefits to experiencing dangerous medical problems. Any substance that is strong enough to help is strong enough to harm, particularly if you don't take it correctly. This goes for the medications your doctor prescribes as well as the medications and nutritional supplements you can buy without a doctor's prescription.

When talk turns to medication, you should tell your doctor if you are pregnant or allergic to any medications, drink alcohol, have health problems other than your arthritis, or take other prescription medications.

To make the most of your medication and for safety's sake, you should ask your doctor the following questions about any medication he or she prescribes:

What is the name of the medication? It's important to know the medication's name and to make sure the bottle your pharmacist fills has that same name. Because some medications have similar-sounding names, mix-ups can occur.

Are there special instructions for taking the drug? Some drugs must be taken with food to minimize stomach distress, while others must be taken on an empty stomach to be absorbed properly. Some drugs must be taken at the same time every day, while other medications may be taken as needed.

How long will it be before I notice effects? If you're expecting to feel better by tomorrow, but the medication your doctor prescribed takes a month to produce any benefits, you need to know. On the other hand, if a medication is made to work quickly, there is no reason to continue taking it for months on end if you're not noticing any results.

What should I do if I miss a dose? No matter how conscientious you are about taking your medication, the time probably will come when you discover that you forgot to take a dose. What do you do? For most drugs, your doctor probably will recommend taking the missed dose as soon as you realize your error, and then resuming your regular schedule. If a lot of time has passed, however, it may be best to skip the missed dose and resume your medication with the next scheduled dose. If you're in doubt, it's always best to ask your doctor or pharmacist.

What should I do if I experience side effects? Although an adverse reaction may be sufficient reason to stop taking one drug immediately, abruptly stopping another one could be dangerous. Find out which side effects are likely to pass, which reactions may warrant a call to the doctor's office and which require immediate attention from a physician or other health-care professional.

Is a generic available? As discussed, a generic medication offers the same results as a brandname medication, for less money. If a generic is available, you may want to try it. In some states, your physician's prescription pad will have a place to check if a generic drug is an acceptable alternative for your particular condition.

Is there anything else I should know about taking this medicine? Now is the time to address any other concerns you might have. For example, if you have trouble swallowing pills, make sure the medication you are taking can be crushed and mixed with liquid. Some cannot; ask your pharmacist. If the drug your doctor prescribes is one of them, you'll need to ask for a medication that can be injected or that comes in a liquid solution.

If you still have questions about the medications your doctor prescribes, ask for pamphlets or brochures that might help, or contact your local Arthritis Foundation office for brochures on arthritis medications. Drug manufacturers' Web sites also offer information about their drugs. For general questions or concerns about medications, the sources listed in Chapter 4 may help.

In Chapter 6, we'll discuss some of the specific types of drugs your doctor might prescribe for your arthritis.

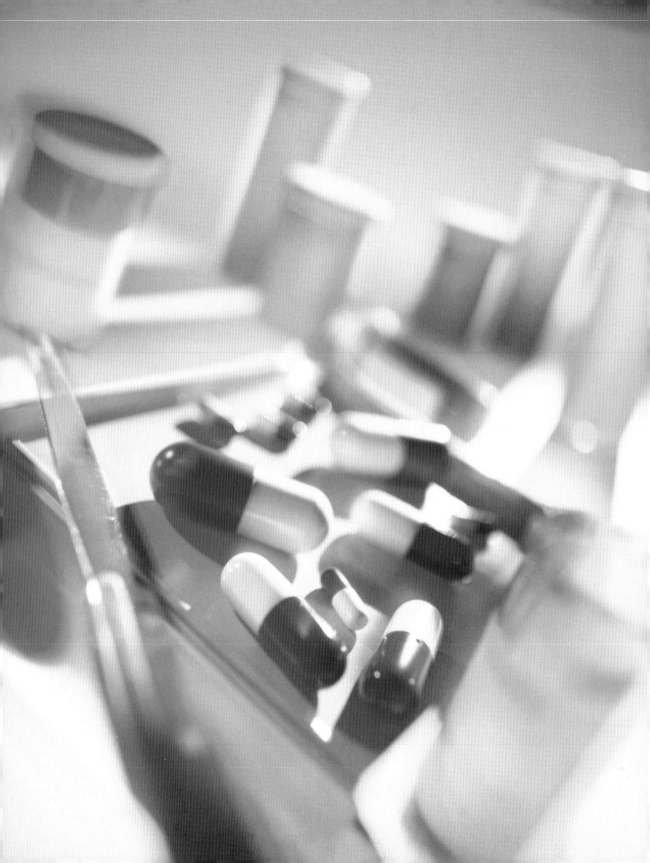

Common Arthritis Drugs

6

CHAPTER 6:
COMMON ARTHRITIS DRUGS

As we discussed in Chapter 5, medications are likely to be a part of almost any arthritis treatment plan. The medications available today can, in many cases, ease pain, relieve inflammation, prevent dangerous disease complications, strengthen porous bone, lessen flares and slow, stop or even prevent joint damage.

In this chapter, we'll discuss some of the specific types of medications used in the treatment of arthritis and related conditions. The particular disease you have, as well as its symptoms and its severity, will dictate the type of medication your doctor prescribes. Some types of medications are used to treat a wide variety of diseases, while other treatments are unique for certain diseases.

Following are some of the medications that may be a part of your arthritis treatment plan.

NONSTEROIDAL ANTI-INFLAMMATORY DRUGS (NSAIDs)

No matter what form of arthritis you have, there's a pretty good chance that the first drug your doctor prescribes or recommends will be a nonsteroidal anti-inflammatory drug (NSAID). The chances are that you already have taken such drugs on your own.

The class of drugs called NSAIDs includes one of the oldest and most widely used medications, aspirin, as well as the popular over-the-counter medications ibuprofen (*Advil, Motrin IB, Nuprin*), ketoprofen (*Actron, Orudis KT*)

and naproxen sodium (*Aleve*), which are available in higher doses by prescription. About a dozen other NSAIDs are available only by prescription.

All NSAIDs ease pain and inflammation by blocking the production of bodily chemicals called prostaglandins, which also play a role in numerous other bodily functions, including blood clotting, menstrual cramps, labor contractions and kidney function. The specific NSAID your doctor prescribes will depend on a number of factors, including the following:

Your doctors' familiarity with the drugs. Because there are so many different NSAIDs, most doctors select four or five that can be used for all patients.

What works best for you. For unknown reasons, some people seem to do better on certain NSAIDs than others. If your first – or second or third – NSAID doesn't significantly improve pain and inflammation, your doctor may try another.

Convenience. Some NSAIDs come in once-a-day formulations. If you prefer the convenience of taking just one pill a day, ask your doctor to prescribe that type. Be aware, however, that once-a-day medications are not the best option for all people. Because they stay in the body longer than drugs designed to be taken more frequently, they may not be safe for people whose bodies have trouble metabolizing the drugs or for those who are at increased risk of side effects.

Economics. Let's face it, some NSAIDs (particularly the ones that are available as generics) cost less than others. Some insurance carriers may pay for only certain NSAIDs. When all other factors are equal or similar, you probably will prefer the NSAID that your insurance covers or that will be least expensive.

Ulcer risk. One of the biggest factors in determining which NSAID your doctor will prescribe is whether you have had ulcers or at increased risk of getting them. Taking NSAIDs, particularly for a long period and at high doses, can lead to gastric distress and bleeding. This effect is caused by prostaglandins, the pain- and inflammation-causing chemicals that NSAIDs inhibit. Prostaglandins have other functions in the body, including protecting the stomach lining from its own gastric juices. When prostaglandins are hindered, so is that protection. If ulcers are a problem or a potential problem, your doctor may prescribe one of the following drugs:

- **COX-2 inhibitors.** One of the newest additions to arthritis treatment, these are a class of NSAIDs that reduce pain and inflammation without increasing the stomach's vulnerability to damage. Celecoxib (*Celebrex*) and rofecoxib (*Vioxx*) work by selectively inhibiting cyclooxygenase-2 (COX-2), the enzyme that is responsible for production of inflammatory prostaglandins involved in arthritis,

without interfering with COX-1, a similar enzyme that is responsible for the production of prostaglandins that protect the stomach.

- **Diclofenac and misoprostol.** Marketed under the name *Arthrotec*, this formulation combines the NSAID diclofenac with a synthetic prostaglandin to replace the stomach-protecting prostaglandins that the NSAID inhibits.

- **Nonacetylated salicylates.** Chemically related to aspirin, these drugs are formulated to be easier on the stomach than aspirin or traditional NSAIDs. Nonacetylated salicylates include such drugs as choline and magnesium salicylates (*CMT, Tricosal, Trilisate*), choline salicylate (*Arthropan*), and magnesium salicylate (*Magan, Mobidin, Mobogesic*).

- **Other NSAIDs.** Other types of NSAIDs that might be easier on the stomach include buffered tablets, enteric-coated tablets that don't dissolve until they reach the small intestine, and time-released capsules or tablets that release the drug slowly into the bloodstream.

ANALGESICS

If your arthritis causes pain, you may benefit from an analgesic, or pain-relieving, medication. Analgesic medications are prescribed purely for pain relief – that is, they don't work against inflammation the way NSAIDs do.

The most commonly used and readily available analgesic is acetaminophen (*Tylenol*). Based on its cost, effectiveness and safety, the American

WHEN NSAIDs CAUSE STOMACH DISTRESS

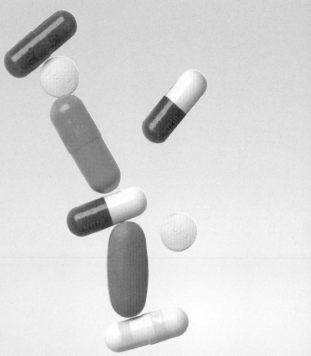

Any time you take a medication, you open yourself to the risk of side effects. If you're among the millions of Americans who take nonsteroidal anti-inflammatory drugs (NSAIDs), the drugs prescribed most commonly for arthritis inflammation and pain and fever from other causes, the most likely side effects will involve your stomach.

Because traditional NSAIDs inhibit the body's production of prostaglandins, hormone-like substances that protect the stomach lining, using these drugs can lead to problems ranging from occasional nausea and heartburn to bleeding ulcers.

Fortunately, there are ways to minimize these risks. The most notable method is using one of the new COX-2 inhibitors, which are NSAIDs that are designed to ease pain and inflammation without interfering with stomach protection. COX-2s aren't the whole or only answer to NSAID-related stomach problems. Here are some others:

Replacing prostaglandins. In 1989, a synthetic prostaglandin called misoprostol (*Cytotec*) was approved by the FDA. By replacing the stomach's natural protective prostaglandins, misoprostol can reduce the risk of new ulcers or promote the healing of existing ulcers. One product, approved in recent years, combines the NSAID diclofenac sodium with misoprostol. Marketed under the name *Arthrotec*, the drug is available only by prescription.

Blocking stomach acid. Because neither COX-2s nor misoprostol reduce the risk of other gastrointestinal side effects (in fact, misoprostol is associated with increased abdominal pain and diarrhea), if you have a problem with NSAID-related indigestion, heartburn or nausea, you may benefit from taking another medication with your NSAID. Drugs that might be helpful come from two categories – histamine blockers (or H2 blockers) and proton pump inhibitors – along with traditional NSAIDs. Both types of drugs work by reducing the amount of acid produced in the stomach. Histamine blockers include such drugs as cimetidine (*Tagamet*), ranitidine hydrochloride (*Zantac*), famotidine (*Pepcid*) and nizatidine (*Axid Pulvules*). Proton pump inhibitors include omeprazole (*Prilosec*) and lansoprazole (*Prevacid*). Neither proton pump inhibitors nor H2 blockers decrease the risk of GI bleeding.

Although several of these drugs have become available over the counter, you should always check with your doctor before taking one of them with NSAIDs. One study suggested that H2 blockers may mask the early symptoms of stomach ulcers.

Despite the availability of new NSAIDs and medications to ease NSAID-associated stomach problems, the only safe way to prevent NSAID problems is not to take NSAIDs.

For a free copy of the *Arthritis Today Drug Guide*, a complete guide to the most common arthritis drugs, their side effects and dosages, call 800/283-7800 or log on to www.arthritis.org.

College of Rheumatology recommends acetaminophen as a first line of treatment against osteoarthritis pain. For many people, acetaminophen alone is sufficient to ease OA pain.

Acetaminophen can be purchased over the counter under a variety of different trade and store names and often is the active ingredient in products labeled "aspirin-free pain reliever."

Until recently, acetaminophen was the only analgesic used for day-to-day arthritis pain. Although doctors sometimes prescribed narcotic analgesics such as oxycodone (*OxyContin, Roxicodone*) or propoxyphene hydrochloride (*Darvon, PP-Cap*) for arthritis patients, these types of pain relievers traditionally have been used only for the acute pain of surgery or osteoporotic fracture or for severe musculoskeletal pain.

In recent years, however, the medical profession has begun to focus on the importance of treating nonmalignant pain and the unique ability of narcotics to ease pain. In fact, when the American College of Rheumatology revised its guidelines for treating osteoarthritis in 2000, it acknowledged, for the first time, the role of narcotic analgesics in treating osteoarthritis pain. One analgesic, tramadol (*Ultram*), was mentioned specifically in the group's treatment guidelines. Narcotic drugs may carry the risk of dependence, causing some debate on their use for treating the pain associated with a chronic illness (see sidebar).

Because analgesic medications don't influence prostaglandin production the way NSAIDs do, they don't carry NSAIDs' risk of ulcers. They do, however, have side effects of their own, which may include drowsiness, grogginess and the potential for dependence.

TOPICAL OINTMENTS

If you find you can't take oral analgesics or if you have just a few joints or sore muscles that need soothing, you might want to try one of the many analgesic salves, creams, rubs and balms available over the counter. The American College of Rheumatology's recently revised treatment guidelines for OA of the hip and knee acknowledge the role of topical analgesics for OA pain, particularly in people whose pain is mild to moderate and not relieved by acetaminophen alone.

Unlike most other arthritis medications, which are swallowed or injected, these preparations work on the area into which you rub them, minimizing the risk of systemic side effects.

The effects of topical analgesics come from one or more active ingredients. Here are some of the most common ones:

Capsaicin. A highly purified natural ingredient found in cayenne peppers, capsaicin works by depleting the amount of a neurotransmitter called substance P that is believed to send pain messages to the brain. For the first couple of weeks of use, the ingredient may cause burning or stinging. Capsaicin is available under the product names *Zostrix*, *Zostrix HP*,

Capzasin-P and others. Menthacin includes both capsaicin and counterirritants.

Counterirritants. Like stepping on your toe to take your mind off a headache, counterirritants stimulate or irritate the nerve endings to distract the brain's attention from musculoskeletal pain. Counterirritants encompass such substances as menthol, oil of wintergreen, camphor, eucalyptus oil, turpentine oil, dihydrochloride and methyl nicotinate and are found in such products as *ArthriCare*, *Eucalyptamint*, *Icy Hot* and *Therapeutic Mineral Ice*.

Salicylates. Like the salicylates found in many oral pain relievers, these compounds may work by inhibiting prostaglandins. In topical preparations, they act as counterirritants, stimulating or irritating nerve endings. Brand-name examples of topical analgesics containing salicylates include *Aspercreme*, *Ben-Gay*, *Flexall*, *Mobisyl* and *Sportscreme*.

GLUCOCORTICOIDS

If you have an inflammatory disease, such as rheumatoid arthritis, lupus, polymyalgia rheumatica, polymyositis or an arthritis-related condition called giant cell arteritis, there's a good chance that your doctor will prescribe a glucocorticoid medication for you. Glucocorticoids are potent fighters of inflammation. They can help reduce harmful joint inflammation and control destructive inflammation of the kidneys, blood vessels and other organs.

The most-prescribed glucocorticoid for arthritis-related diseases is prednisone (*Deltasone*,

The Narcotics Debate

Some doctors would never prescribe narcotics for arthritis or a related chronic disease. Others argue that they can be an appropriate drug for pain relief and promoting sleep. Even doctors who support their use agree that narcotics are only necessary for a small number of people, and then only in tandem with a comprehensive treatment program.

If pain relief is not achieved with NSAIDs, tricyclics, acetaminophen or tramadol, then narcotics such as codeine, hydrocodone, oxycodone or methadone may be considered. The decision to go this route requires patient counseling on dependency and expected side effects. Most physicians will require their patients to sign a contract that outlines appropriate use of the drugs and the physician's expectations regarding ongoing use. Below are what many doctors view as central issues in the debate:

Advantages:

- Narcotics are the most effective available medications for managing pain.
- The majority of arthritis patients don't need narcotics. But those that do should have the option for a trial period.
- The addiction rate from narcotics is one percent. Addiction (compulsive, self-destructive use) is not the same as dependence (withdrawal symptoms if the drug is stopped abruptly).
- Less pain results in better functioning.

Disadvantages:

- When you use narcotics, you are treating pain solely as a symptom, without necessarily eliminating the factors that cause it. Therefore, narcotics should be used only in the context of a thorough medical management program.
- Dependence is an expected result of treatment.
- Narcotics will dull pain, but not eliminate it. In other words, they are not a "cure" for the pain associated with arthritis or related conditions.
- Tolerance to narcotics occurs after a time – from months to years – so that increasing the dosage is necessary to maintain the same level of response.
- Narcotics have side effects such as mental fuzziness, constipation and nausea.

Orasone, Prednicen-M, Sterapred), but there are several others, including cortisone (*Cortone Acetate*), prednisolone (*Prelone*) and methylprednisolone (*Medrol*).

Glucocorticoids may be taken systemically, in pill form or by injection into a vein or muscle. If you have just one or a few inflamed joints, however, your doctor may inject a glucocorticoid compound directly into the joints for quick, temporary relief without wide-ranging side effects. Glucocorticoids also are available to treat arthritis-related rashes or psoriasis lesions.

When used in high doses or long-term, glucocorticoids are associated with a number of side effects, including Cushing's syndrome (weight gain, "moon" face, thin skin, muscle weakness, brittle bones), cataracts, hypertension, increased appetite, elevated blood sugar, indigestion, insomnia, mood changes, nervousness and restlessness. Those risks can be minimized by using the lowest doses that control your disease.

Some doctors reduce the risk of glucocorticoid side effects by prescribing alternate-day therapy (that is, you take your dose every other day, instead of every day).

DISEASE-MODIFYING ANTI-RHEUMATIC DRUGS (DMARDs)

Disease-modifying antirheumatic drugs (DMARDs) are a class of medications that doctors prescribe for rheumatoid arthritis and other inflammatory forms of arthritis, such as psoriatic arthritis or ankylosing spondylitis. As the name suggests, DMARDs actually modify the course of disease, slowing or even stopping its progression. Most of these drugs work by suppressing the immune system, which is involved in the joint damage that occurs in RA and other diseases.

If your doctor prescribes a disease-modifying antirheumatic drug, don't expect quick results. These drugs often take several weeks or months to produce effects, although most people find the results well worth the wait.

Not too many years ago, if you had seen a doctor about rheumatoid arthritis, he probably wouldn't have prescribed a DMARD – at least not until all other drug options had been exhausted. That approach began to change a decade or so ago, as studies showed that irreparable joint damage often occurs early in the course of disease and that by prescribing DMARDs early on, doctors may be able to get the disease under control before such damage occurs. Doctors also are prescribing more combinations of DMARDs and finding that, for many patients, drug combinations provide benefits that a single drug can't offer.

In 1998, a drug called leflunomide (*Arava*) became one of just a few DMARDs developed specifically for rheumatoid arthritis.

Most DMARDs originally were used and approved for other medical conditions. Methotrexate, for example, originally was a cancer treatment. Cyclosporine (*Neoral, Sandimmune*) was used to prevent organ rejection in people who had undergone transplants, and hydroxychloroquine sulfate (*Plaquenil*) was used to treat malaria. It was only after years of use for these other conditions that these DMARDs were approved for rheumatic diseases.

Despite the drugs developed in recent years, existing DMARDs continue to play an important role in managing rheumatoid arthritis. Methotrexate (*Rheumatrex, Trexall*), for example, is considered by many rheumatologists to be the "gold standard" for RA treatment. Other DMARDs, including oral or injectable gold, are used much less frequently than they once were.

BIOLOGIC RESPONSE MODIFIERS

Unlike traditional DMARDs, which may cause widespread suppression of the immune system, biologic response modifiers (BRMs, or biologic agents) target specific immune system components, such as chemical messengers called cytokines, that play a role in the inflammation and damage of the disease.

The two currently available agents, etanercept (*Enbrel*) and infliximab (*Remicade*), use different chemical actions to block an inflammatory cytokine called tumor necrosis factor (TNF), which is believed to play a role in RA and some other diseases. As a result, these agents retard the inflammatory response and ease the signs and symptoms of RA. However, ongoing research has shown that their effects go beyond symptomatic relief; both inhibit the progression of structural damage in patients with moderate to severely active rheumatoid arthritis. (Infliximab is approved for use in conjunction with methotrexate.) While some doctors reserve biologic agents for patients whose arthritis hasn't responded well to more conventional therapies, others are starting to prescribe them earlier in the disease process in an effort to ward off or reduce permanent joint damage.

One disadvantage of both agents is that they must be injected. Etanercept is injected twice a week through a small needle just beneath the skin. Infliximab is administered intravenously every eight weeks in a two-hour outpatient procedure. For most people, the biggest drawback of biologic agents is the cost. A year's supply of etanercept costs approximately $11,000, and infliximab costs approximately $1,222 for each eight-week dose plus the cost of the infusion. (Actual dose, and therefore, cost, is based on body weight.)

Other biologic agents in testing and development target other chemicals. One of the most promising is anakinra (*Kineret*), an agent that inhibits the action of an inflammatory cytokine called interleukin-1 (IL-1) and that may receive FDA approval as early as late 2001.

Some biologic agents in development target more than one chemical. Some are being designed so that they can be taken orally.

MEDICATIONS FOR OSTEOPOROSIS

Just a decade ago, women had only two options when it came to preventing osteoporosis: take estrogen replacement therapy or take their chances. For men at risk of the brittle-bone disease, even estrogen wasn't an option.

Today, however, there are an increasing number of options for women who have or are at risk of developing osteoporotic fractures. And in 2000, a drug called alendronate (*Fosamax*) became the first medication approved by the FDA for treating osteoporosis in men.

Medications for osteoporosis prevention or treatment fall into the following general categories. Whichever treatment your doctor prescribes, ask about the advisability of taking calcium and vitamin D supplements. See "Nutrition for Healthy Bones" on page 71 for more information on calcium and vitamin D.

Hormones

Estrogen. The most widely used osteoporosis medication for post-menopausal women is the female hormone estrogen (*Premarin, Estratab, Menest*). Before menopause, high levels of estrogen in the body help keep bone strong by causing the death of cells that are responsible for bone degradation. For women who have not had a hysterectomy, doctors prescribe estrogen in combination with the hormone progesterone (*Premphase, Prempro*) to minimize any risks of estrogen on the uterus. If you are going through menopause and experiencing troublesome hot flashes and other symptoms, estrogen replacement can ease those symptoms as well as bone loss.

Calcitonin. Another hormone used to treat osteoporosis is calcitonin, which is similar to a hormone produced by our parathyroid glands (two pairs of endocrine glands that are situated behind or within the thyroid gland). Parathyroid hormone occurs naturally in the body, controls the distribution of calcium and phosphate, and has been shown to have an effect on bone growth. Calcitonin, which is administered by injection (*Calcimar, Miacalcin*) or nasal spray (*Miacalcin*), has been shown to reduce fracture risk. It also has some pain-relieving effects for people who already have had fractures.

Bisphosphonates

A class of medication used in the treatment of bone diseases, including the arthritis-related condition Paget's disease, bisphosphonates are used increasingly in the treatment of osteoporosis because they inhibit bone resorption. In recent years, two bisphosphonate medications, alendronate (*Fosamax*) and risedronate sodium (*Actonel*), were approved for osteoporosis. Risedronate sodium is approved specifically for glucocorticoid-induced osteoporosis. Unlike many of the other medications used for osteoporosis, bisphosphonates are appropriate for men.

Selective Estrogen Receptor Molecules

One of the newest classes of medications for osteoporosis, selective estrogen receptor molecules (SERMs), including raloxifene hydrochloride (*Evista*), work much like estrogen to slow bone loss. The biggest difference is that they lack some of estrogen's side effects, mainly those related to breast and uterine tissue, making them an attractive alternative to estrogen replacement for women at increased risk of breast or uterine cancer.

MEDICATIONS FOR FIBROMYALGIA

Although there aren't any drugs approved specifically for fibromyalgia, if you have the condition, you may benefit from some of the drugs used for arthritis pain – namely, NSAIDs or analgesics. Your doctor also may prescribe some medications that aren't commonly used in other forms of arthritis or related conditions.

Because studies have shown that lack of deep, restorative sleep is a common problem in people with fibromyalgia and that poor sleep quality contributes to the condition's characteristic muscle pain, fatigue and concentration difficulties, some of the most popular medications are those that promote deep sleep. These drugs include:

Antidepressants. When administered in smaller doses than those used to treat depression, antidepressant medications, including tricyclics – amitriptyline hydrochloride (*Elavil, Endep*), doxepin (*Adapin, Sinequan*) and nortriptyline (*Aventyl, Pamelor*) – and selective serotonin reuptake inhibitors (SSRIs) – fluoxetine (*Prozac*), paroxetine (*Paxil*) and sertraline (*Zoloft*) – may help people with fibromyalgia get the restorative sleep they need.

Although tricyclic antidepressants usually are the medications of choice for fibromyalgia-related sleep problems, research suggests that combining low doses of tricyclic antidepressants with SSRIs may increase each drug's benefits to people with fibromyalgia

Muscle relaxants. Muscle-relaxing medications, such as cyclobenzaprine (*Cycloflex, Flexeril*), may help reduce muscle spasms associated with fibromyalgia and help induce deep sleep.

Anti-anxiety medications. Like antidepressants, anti-anxiety medications, such as temazepam (*Restoril*), may be given in low doses to promote sleep. Some doctors believe these drugs work by interfering with brain-wave activity that keeps people with fibromyalgia in a superficial stage of sleep.

Other fibromyalgia treatments. Some of the newest sleep aids promise to be effective for people with fibromyalgia. These drugs include zolpidem (*Ambien*) and zaleplon (*Sonata*).

MEDICATIONS FOR GOUT

Whether you have had one gout attack or ten, chances are you that would do just about anything to keep from having another. Fortunately, there are medications that can ease or prevent future attacks. Determining which medication is right for you requires an understanding of the underlying problem.

Gout is caused when excess uric acid builds up in the body and is deposited as crystals in body tissues, including the joints and skin. If you have gout because your body produces too much uric acid, a drug called allopurinol (*Lopurin, Zyloprim*) will slow the rate of uric acid production and help prevent future attacks. On the other hand, if the build-up is related to your body's inability to excrete uric acid properly, two other drugs – probenecid (*Benemid, Probalan*) or sulfinpyrazone (*Anturane*) – may help prevent attacks by increasing the amount of uric acid passed in the urine.

Although preventing attacks is a goal for anyone with gout, medications used to prevent gout attacks do little, if anything, to ease an attack once it has started. Ironically, any of these drugs may, at first, cause an increase in gout attacks, as the body mobilizes uric acid. For that reason, your doctor should prescribe an NSAID or anti-inflammatory drug called colchicine along with these uric acid regulators to ease the pain and inflammation of attacks. Once an attack has started, NSAIDs or glucocorticoids can provide symptomatic relief for gout.

WHERE TO LEARN MORE

To learn more about the drugs you take, you may want to check some of these other resources. Some are meant for physicians, but you may wish to know more about your drugs than pharmacy inserts provide.

Books

United States Pharmacopeia Dispensing Information (USP DI) Volume II Advice for the Patient, Drug Information in Lay Language. (2001, Micromedex, $75.) Offers easy-to-understand information about more than 11,000 brand-name and generic medications marketed in the United States and Canada. To order, call 800/877-6209 or visit the Micro-medex Web site at www.micromedex.com/products.

Physician's Desk Reference (PDR). (2001, Medical Economics, $77.95.) Features up-to-date FDA-approved information on more than 4,000 prescription drugs, and photos of the most prescribed drugs. To order, call 800/232-7379 or visit the Medical Economics Web site at www.medec.com/html/products.

PDR for Nonprescription Drugs and Dietary Supplements. (2001, Medical Economics $48.95.) Contains detailed descriptions of the most commonly used nonprescription drugs and preparations, along with full-color photographs of hundreds of over-the-counter drugs for quick identification. To order, call 800/232-7379 or visit the Medical Economics Web site at www.medec.com/html/products.

Web Sites

www.OnHealth.com/conditions/resources/pharmacy/index.asp offers clear information on thousands of prescription and over-the-counter medications, listed by generic and brand name. This site also features a tool that allows you to check for drugs that interact with one another.

www.safemedication.com, a Web site of the American Health-System Pharmacists, offers important information on using medications safely and wisely.

www.FDA.gov, the Web site of the Food and Drug Administration, offers a search engine for looking up information about medications and numerous food- and drug-related subjects.

NUTRITION FOR HEALTHY BONES

Whether you have osteoporosis or want to prevent it, it's essential that you get plenty of the bone-building mineral calcium. Calcium is available in dairy products, canned sardines or salmon with bones, fortified juices and green, leafy vegetables.

Vitamin D also is needed to help your body use the calcium you consume. Dietary sources of vitamin D include fortified milk or dairy products, fortified breakfast cereals, egg yolks and fatty fish.

Following are the Reference Daily Intakes (RDIs) established by the Institute of Medicine for calcium and vitamin D. As these lists show, requirements for the two nutrients vary with age. Consult your doctor or nutritionist to learn more.

Daily Calcium Requirement

1-3 years	500 mg
4-8 years	800 mg
9-18 years	1,300 mg
19-50 years	1,000 mg
51 years and older	1,200 mg
PREGNANT OR BREASTFEEDING	
14-18 years	1,300 mg
19-50 years	1,000 mg

Daily Vitamin D Requirement

1 to 50 years	200 international units (IUs)
51 to 70 years	400 IUs
over 70 years	600 IUs

If you live in a northern climate with limited exposure to full sun, or if you routinely wear sunscreen, your body may not make the amount of vitamin D it needs. Likewise, you may not be consuming enough vitamin D- and calcium-rich foods. If you think that you might not be getting enough of either nutrient, speak to your doctor or a dietitian about calcium and vitamin D supplements.

Some medications, particularly the newer ones, have their own Web sites. For example: www.Synvisc.com, www.Hyalgan.com, www. Enbrel.com, www.remicade.com, www.arava. com, www.Celebrex.com and www.Vioxx.com.

Other Sources of Information

The Arthritis Foundation. In addition to the comprehensive *Arthritis Today Drug Guide*, the Arthritis Foundation offers free single copies of brochures about numerous arthritis medications. To inquire about a specific brochure, contact your local Arthritis Foundation office or call 800/283-7800. You also can search the Arthritis Foundation Web site for general information at www.arthritis.org.

Pharmacy handouts. Most pharmacies include a printout with each prescription that tells you how to take the medication, informs you of possible side effects, and advises you about what to do if you experience side effects. Read and become familiar with the information before starting your course of medication, and be sure to discuss any concerns with your doctor or pharmacist.

Package labels and inserts. Each medication, over-the-counter or prescription, comes from the manufacturer with a package insert detailing how the medication should be taken, who should and shouldn't take it, how it works and the side effects associated with it. Inserts can be found in over-the-counter medication packages. For most prescription medications, you will never see the package insert unless you ask for it.

Your physician and pharmacist. If you have any questions about a medication, how it works, or how to take it, the best thing to do is ask your physician or your pharmacist. Ask your doctor any questions about side effects or how to take the medication when he or she is filling out the prescription, or ask your pharmacist when you go to the store to have the prescription filled.

Drugs Used in Treating Arthritis

NSAIDS: NONSTEROIDAL ANTI-INFLAMMATORY DRUGS

NOTE: Possible side effects for all NSAIDs, except where noted, include abdominal pain, dizziness, drowsiness, fluid retention, gastric ulcers and bleeding, greater susceptibility to bruising or bleeding from cuts, heartburn, indigestion, lightheadedness, nausea, nightmares, rash, ringing in the ears, reduction in kidney function, increase in liver enzymes.

Ulcers or internal bleeding can occur without warning. If you consume more than three alcoholic drinks per day, check with your doctor before using these products.

Aspirin
BRAND NAMES: *Anacin, Ascriptin, Bayer, Bufferin, Ecotrin, Excedrin Tablets, ZORprin*, others
DOSAGE: 3,600 to 5,400 mg per day in several doses

Choline and magnesium salicylates
BRAND NAMES: *CMT, Tricosal, Trilisate*
DOSAGE: 2,000 to 3,000 mg per day in 2 or 3 doses
OTHER POSSIBLE SIDE EFFECTS: Bloating, confusion, deafness, diarrhea

Choline salicylate
BRAND NAME: *Arthropan*
DOSAGE: 3,480 to 6,960 mg per day in several doses
OTHER POSSIBLE SIDE EFFECTS: Bloating, confusion, deafness, diarrhea

Diclofenac potassium
BRAND NAME: *Cataflam*
OA DOSAGE: 100 to 150 mg per day in 2 or 3 doses
RA DOSAGE: 100 to 200 mg per day in 3 or 4 doses

Diclofenac sodium
BRAND NAME: *Voltaren*
OA DOSAGE: 100 to 200 mg per day in 2 or 3 doses
RA DOSAGE: 150 to 200 mg per day in 3 or 4 doses

Diclofenac sodium with misoprostol
BRAND NAME: *Arthrotec*
OA DOSAGE: 150 mg per day in 3 doses
RA DOSAGE: 150 to 200 mg per day in 2 to 4 doses

Drugs Used in Treating Arthritis

Diflunisal
BRAND NAME: *Dolobid*
DOSAGE: 500 to 1,500 mg per day in 2 doses

Etodolac
BRAND NAMES: *Lodine, Lodine XL*
DOSAGE: 800 to 1,200 mg per day in 2 to 4 doses for Lodines
400 to 1,000 mg per day in a single dose for Lodine XL

Fenoprofen calcium
BRAND NAME: *Nalfon*
DOSAGE: 900 to 2,400 mg per day in 3 or 4 doses; never more than 3,200 mg per day

Flurbiprofen
BRAND NAME: *Ansaid*
DOSAGE: 200 to 300 mg per day in 2 to 4 doses

Ibuprofen
BRAND NAMES: *Advil, Motrin, Motrin IB, Mediprin, Nuprin*
DOSAGE: 1,200 to 3,200 mg per day in 3 or 4 doses for prescription-strength *Motrin*;
200 to 400 mg every 4 to 6 hours as needed, not exceeding 1,200 mg per day, for
over-the-counter brands.

Indomethacin
BRAND NAME: *Indocin, Indocin SR*
DOSAGE: 50 to 200 mg per day in 2 to 4 doses for *Indocin*; 75 mg per day in 1 dose,
or 150 mg per day in 2 doses, for *Indocin SR*.
OTHER POSSIBLE SIDE EFFECTS: Depression, headache, "spacey" feeling

Ketoprofen
BRAND NAMES: *Actron, Orudis, Orudis KT, Oruvail*
DOSAGE: 200 to 225 mg per day in 3 or 4 doses for *Orudis*; 200 mg per day in 1 dose
for *Oruvail*; 12.5 mg every 4 to 6 hours as needed for *Actron* and *Orudis KT*.

Magnesium salicylate
BRAND NAMES: *Magan, Doan's Pills, Mobidin*
DOSAGE: 2,600 to 4,800 mg per day in 3 to 6 doses
OTHER POSSIBLE SIDE EFFECTS: Bloating, confusion, deafness, diarrhea

Drugs Used in Treating Arthritis

Meclofenamate sodium
BRAND NAME: *Meclomen*
DOSAGE: 200 to 400 mg per day in 4 doses

Mefenamic acid
BRAND NAME: *Ponstel*
DOSAGE: 250 mg every 6 hours as needed, for up to 7 days

Meloxicam
BRAND NAME: *Mobic*
DOSAGE: 7.5 to 15 mg per day in 1 dose

Nabumetone
BRAND NAME: *Relafen*
DOSAGE: 1,000 mg per day in 1 or 2 doses; 2,000 mg per day in 2 doses

Naproxen
BRAND NAMES: *Naprosyn, Naprelan*
DOSAGE: 500 to 1,500 mg per day in 2 doses for *Naprosyn*, 750 or 1,000 mg per day in a single dose for *Naprelan*

Naproxen sodium
BRAND NAMES: *Anaprox, Aleve*
DOSAGE: 550 to 1,650 mg per day in 2 doses for *Anaprox*, 220 mg every 8 to 12 hours as needed for *Aleve*

Oxaprozin
BRAND NAME: *Daypro*
DOSAGE: 1,200 mg per day in 1 or 2 doses or 1,800 mg per day in 2 or 3 doses

Piroxicam
BRAND NAME: *Feldene*
DOSAGE: 20 mg per day in 2 or 3 doses

Salsalate
BRAND NAMES: *Disalcid, Mono-Gesic, Salflex, Salsitab, Amigesic, Anaflex 750, Marthritic*
DOSAGE: 1,000 to 3,000 mg per day in 2 or 3 doses
OTHER POSSIBLE SIDE EFFECTS: Bloating, confusion, deafness, diarrhea

Drugs Used in Treating Arthritis

Sodium salicylate
BRAND NAME: None, generic only
DOSAGE: 3,600 to 5,400 mg per day in several doses
OTHER POSSIBLE SIDE EFFECTS: Bloating, confusion, deafness, diarrhea

Sulindac
BRAND NAME: *Clinoril*
DOSAGE: 300 to 400 mg per day in 2 doses

Tolmetin sodium
BRAND NAME: *Tolectin*
DOSAGE: 1,200 to 1,800 mg per day in 3 doses

COX-2 INHIBITORS

NOTE: This new class of NSAIDs blocks the prostaglandins involved in inflammation, but not the prostaglandins that protect the stomach lining. Therefore, COX-2 inhibitors may not have the stomach-related side effects of traditional NSAIDs. They also may not provide the same protection against heart attacks and strokes.

Celecoxib
BRAND NAME: *Celebrex*
OA DOSAGE: 200 mg per day in 1 or 2 doses
RA DOSAGE: 200 to 400 mg per day in 2 doses
POSSIBLE SIDE EFFECTS: Same as other NSAIDs, except less likely to cause gastric ulcers and susceptibility to bruising and bleeding

Rofecoxib
BRAND NAME: *Vioxx*
OA DOSAGE: 12.5 or 25 mg per day in a single dose
POSSIBLE SIDE EFFECTS: Same as other NSAIDs, except less likely to cause gastric ulcers and susceptibility to bruising and bleeding

Drugs Used in Treating Arthritis

ANALGESICS

These are drugs used for pain relief of arthritis and related conditions.

Acetaminophen
BRAND NAMES: *Anacin* (aspirin-free), *Excedrin caplets, Panadol, Tylenol*
DOSAGE: 325 to 1,000 mg every 4 to 6 hours as needed, no more than 4,000 mg per day
POSSIBLE SIDE EFFECTS: When taken as prescribed, no side effects associated.

Acetaminophen with codeine
BRAND NAMES: *Fioricet, Phenaphen* with codeine, *Tylenol* with codeine
DOSAGE: 15 to 60 mg codeine every 4 hours as needed
POSSIBLE SIDE EFFECTS: Constipation, dizziness or lightheadedness, drowsiness, nausea, unusual tiredness or weakness, vomiting

Hydrocodone with acetaminophen
BRAND NAMES: *Dolacet, Hydrocet, Lorcet, Lortab, Vicodin*
DOSAGE: 2.5 to 10 mg every 4 to 6 hours as needed
POSSIBLE SIDE EFFECTS: Dizziness, drowsiness, lightheadedness, nausea or vomiting, unusual tiredness or weakness

Propoxyphene hydrochloride
BRAND NAMES: *Darvon, PP-Cap, Wygesic*
DOSAGE: 65 mg every 4 hours as needed, no more than 390 mg per day
POSSIBLE SIDE EFFECTS: Dizziness or lightheadedness, drowsiness, nausea and vomiting

Tramadol
BRAND NAME: *Ultram*
DOSAGE: 50 to 100 mg every 6 hours as needed
POSSIBLE SIDE EFFECTS: Dizziness, nausea, constipation, headache, sleepiness

Drugs Used in Treating Arthritis

TOPICAL ANALGESICS

Topical analgesics are salves, creams and rubs that are applied directly to the skin on the painful area. Topical analgesics should never be taken internally. If you are allergic to aspirin, do not use any topical analgesics containing salicylates, which contain the same medication as aspirin. Never use any topical analgesic in conjunction with a heating pad, because deep burns could result. Read brands' labels for specific dosage information.

Counterirritants
BRAND NAMES: *ArthriCare, Eucalyptamint, Icy Hot, Therapeutic Mineral Ice*

Salicylates
BRAND NAMES: *Aspercreme, BenGay, Flexall, Mobisyl, Sportscreme*

Capsaicin
BRAND NAMES: *Capzasin-P, Menthacin (also contains counterirritants), Zostrix, Zostrix HP*

VISCOSUPPLEMENTS

In cases of knee osteoarthritis, viscosupplements may be injected directly into the joint to supplement hyaluronic acid, a substance that gives joint fluid its viscosity and that appears to break down in joints with osteoarthritis. These products relieve pain, but it is not known if they will work on other affected joints, or if they have benefits other than pain relief.

Avoid prolonged weight-bearing activities for 48 hours after injection. These products are not recommended for people allergic to bird feathers, bird proteins and/or eggs.

Possible side effects of both products include pain, fluid collection around the knee, swelling, heat and/or redness at the injection site.

Hyaluronate sodium
BRAND NAME: *Hyalgan, Supartz*
DOSAGE: Five 2 ml injections administered one each week for five weeks

Hylan G-F 20
BRAND NAME: *Synvisc*
DOSAGE: Three 2 ml injections administered at regular intervals over 15 days

Drugs Used in Treating Arthritis

GLUCOCORTICOIDS

Also known as corticosteroids, these drugs are inflammation-fighting hormones. The following side effects are possible for all the following glucocorticoids, but are more common with high doses and long-term use:

Cushing's syndrome (weight gain, "moon" face, thin skin, muscle weakness, brittle bones), cataracts, hypertension, increased appetite, elevated blood sugar, indigestion, insomnia, mood changes, nervousness or restlessness. Dosage varies greatly based on disease severity.

Cortisone
BRAND NAMES: *Cortone Acetate*
RA DOSAGE: 5 to 150 mg per day in a single dose

Dexamethasone
BRAND NAMES: *Decadron, Hexadrol*
RA DOSAGE: 0.5 to 9 mg per day in a single dose

Hydrocortisone
BRAND NAMES: *Cortef, Hydrocortone*
RA DOSAGE: 20 to 240 mg per day in a single dose or divided into several doses

Methylprednisolone
BRAND NAME: *Medrol*
RA DOSAGE: 4 to 160 mg per day in a single dose or divided into several doses

Prednisolone
BRAND NAME: *Prelone*
RA DOSAGE: 5 to 200 mg per day in a single dose or divided into several doses

Prednisolone sodium phosphate (liquid only)
BRAND NAME: *Pediapred*
RA DOSAGE: 5 to 60 ml per day in 1 to 3 doses

Prednisone
BRAND NAMES: *Deltasone, Orasone, Prednicen-M, Sterapred*
RA DOSAGE: 1 to 60 mg per day in a single dose or divided into several doses

Drugs Used in Treating Arthritis

Triamcinolone

BRAND NAME: *Aristocort*

RA DOSAGE: 4 to 60 mg per day in a single dose or divided into several doses

BIOLOGIC RESPONSE MODIFIERS

NOTE: This new class of arthritis drugs blocks TNF (tumor necrosis factor), believed to play a major role in causing inflammation and joint damage. They may make patients more susceptible to infections. Little is known about their long-term side effects.

Etanercept

BRAND NAME: *Enbrel*

RA DOSAGE: 25 mg twice per week, given by subcutaneous (beneath the skin) injection

POSSIBLE SIDE EFFECTS: Redness and/or itching, pain or swelling at the injection site

Infliximab

BRAND NAME: *Remicade*

RA DOSAGE: Determined by body weight. Drug is infused intravenously in a two-hour outpatient procedure every 1 to 2 months. Only approved for use in combination with methotrexate in rheumatoid arthritis.

POSSIBLE SIDE EFFECTS: Upper respiratory infection, headache, nausea, coughing

DMARDS – DISEASE-MODIFYING ANTIRHEUMATIC DRUGS – AND OTHERS

NOTE: These drugs modify the course in inflammatory conditions. Minocycline, an antibiotic, is also included here. Many DMARDs are used in combination to increase effectiveness and decrease side effects. Comprehensive explanations of cautions are contained in this chapter.

Auranofin (oral gold)

BRAND NAME: *Ridaura*

RA DOSAGE: 6 to 9 mg per day in 1 or 2 doses

POSSIBLE SIDE EFFECTS: Abdominal or stomach cramps or pain, bloated feeling, decrease in or loss of appetite, diarrhea or loose stools, gas or indigestion, mouth sores, nausea or vomiting, skin rash or itching

Drugs Used in Treating Arthritis

Azathioprine
BRAND NAME: *Imuran*
RA DOSAGE: 50 to 150 mg per day in 1 to 3 doses, based on body weight
POSSIBLE SIDE EFFECTS: Cough, fever and chills, loss of appetite, nausea or vomiting, skin rash, unusual bleeding or bruising, unusual tiredness or weakness

Cyclophosphamide
BRAND NAME: *Cytoxan*
RA DOSAGE: 50 to 150 mg per day in a single dose; may also be given intravenously
POSSIBLE SIDE EFFECTS: Blood in urine or burning on urination, confusion or agitation, cough, dizziness, fever and chills, infertility in men and women, loss of appetite, missed menstrual periods, nausea or vomiting, unusual bleeding or bruising, unusual tiredness or weakness

Cyclosporine
BRAND NAMES: *Sandimmune, Neoral*
RA DOSAGE: 100 to 400 mg per day in 2 doses, based on body weight
POSSIBLE SIDE EFFECTS: Tender or enlarged gums, high blood pressure, increase in hair growth, kidney problems, loss of appetite, tremors

Hydroxychloroquine sulfate
BRAND NAME: *Plaquenil*
RA DOSAGE: 200 to 600 mg per day in 1 or 2 doses
POSSIBLE SIDE EFFECTS: Black spots in visual field, diarrhea, loss of appetite, nausea, rash

Methotrexate
BRAND NAME: *Rheumatrex, Trexall*
RA DOSAGE: 7.5 to 15 mg per week in 3 doses, or 10 mg per week in a single dose; may also be given by injection
POSSIBLE SIDE EFFECTS: Cough, diarrhea, hair loss, loss of appetite, unusual bleeding or bruising, liver toxicity, lung toxicity

Leflunomide
BRAND NAME: *Arava*
RA DOSAGE: 10 to 20 mg per day in a single dose
POSSIBLE SIDE EFFECTS: Diarrhea, skin rash, liver toxicity, hair loss

Drugs Used in Treating Arthritis

Minocycline
BRAND NAME: *Minocin*
RA DOSAGE: 200 mg per day in 2 doses
POSSIBLE SIDE EFFECTS: Dizziness, vaginal infections, nausea, headache, skin rash

Penicillamine
BRAND NAMES: *Cuprimine, Depen*
RA DOSAGE: 125 to 250 mg per day in a single dose to start, increased to not more than 1,500 mg per day in 3 doses
POSSIBLE SIDE EFFECTS: Diarrhea, joint pain, lessening or loss of sense of taste, loss of appetite, fever, hives or itching, mouth sores, nausea or vomiting, skin rash, stomach pain, swollen glands, unusual bleeding or bruising, weakness

Sulfasalazine
BRAND NAME: *Azulfidine, Azulfidine E-N Tabs*
RA DOSAGE: 500mg to 3 grams per day in 2 to 4 doses
POSSIBLE SIDE EFFECTS: Stomach upset, diarrhea, dizziness, headache, light sensitivity, itching, appetite loss, liver abnormalities, lowered blood count, nausea or vomiting, rash

Injectable gold (Gold sodium thiolomate and Aurothioglucose)
BRAND NAMES: Gold sodium thiolomate: *Myochrysine*; Aurothioglucose: *Solganol*
RA DOSAGE: 10 mg in a single dose the first week, 25 mg the following week, then 25 to 50 mg per week thereafter. Frequency may be reduced after several months.
POSSIBLE SIDE EFFECTS: Irritation or soreness of tongue, metallic taste, skin rash or itching, soreness, swelling or bleeding of gums, unusual bleeding or bruising

FIBROMYALGIA DRUGS

At this time, there are no drugs specifically approved by the Food and Drug Administration for treating fibromyalgia. Here are some drugs that may alleviate certain symptoms associated with fibromyalgia, including pain, sleep problems and muscle aches.

Antidepressants
Antidepressants, including tricyclics and selective serotonin reuptake inhibitors (SSRIs), help people with fibromyalgia get the deep, restorative sleep they often lack.

Drugs Used in Treating Arthritis

TRICYCLICS:

Amitriptyline hydrochloride

BRAND NAME: *Elavil, Endep*

DOSAGE: 10 to 50 mg per day in a single dose

POSSIBLE SIDE EFFECTS: Difficulty concentrating, dizziness, drowsiness, dry mouth, headache, increased appetite (including craving for sweets), nausea, sleep disturbances, unpleasant taste, urinary retention, weakness or tiredness, weight gain

Doxepin

BRAND NAME: *Adapin, Sinequan*

DOSAGE: 10 to 100 mg in the morning in a single dose

POSSIBLE SIDE EFFECTS: Difficulty concentrating, dizziness, drowsiness, dry mouth, headache, increased appetite (including craving for sweets), nausea, sleep disturbances, unpleasant taste, urinary retention, weakness or tiredness, weight gain

Nortriptyline

BRAND NAME: *Aventyl, Pamelor*

DOSAGE: 10 to 100 mg in the morning in a single dose

POSSIBLE SIDE EFFECTS: Difficulty concentrating, dizziness, drowsiness, dry mouth, headache, increased appetite (including craving for sweets), nausea, sleep disturbances, unpleasant taste, urinary retention, weakness or tiredness, weight gain

SELECTIVE SEROTONIN REUPTAKE INHIBITORS (SSRIs)

Fluoxetine

BRAND NAME: *Prozac*

DOSAGE: 20 mg per day in a single dose

POSSIBLE SIDE EFFECTS: Anxiety and nervousness, diarrhea, dry mouth, headache, increased sweating, nausea, trouble sleeping

Paroxetine

BRAND NAME: *Paxil*

DOSAGE: 10 mg per day in a single dose

POSSIBLE SIDE EFFECTS: Constipation, decreased sexual ability, dizziness, dry mouth, headache, nausea, difficulty urinating, tremors, trouble sleeping, unusual tiredness or weakness, vomiting

Drugs Used in Treating Arthritis

Sertraline
BRAND NAME: *Zoloft*

DOSAGE: 25 to 50 mg per day in a single dose

POSSIBLE SIDE EFFECTS: Decreased appetite or weight loss; decreased sexual drive or ability; diarrhea; drowsiness; dryness of the mouth; headache, stomach or abdominal cramps, gas or pain; tremors; trouble sleeping; clumsiness or unsteadiness; dizziness or lightheadedness; drowsiness; slurred speech

BENZODIAZEPINES – SLEEP MEDICATION

Temazepam
BRAND NAME: *Restoril*

DOSAGE: 15 mg per day in a single dose

POSSIBLE SIDE EFFECTS: When taken as prescribed, temazepam is not usually associated with side effects.

MUSCLE RELAXANTS

Cyclobenzaprine
BRAND NAMES: *Cycloflex, Flexeril*

DOSAGE: 10 to 30 mg per day in 1 to 3 doses

POSSIBLE SIDE EFFECTS: Dizziness or lightheadedness, drowsiness, dry mouth, confusion

OTHER DRUGS USED FOR FIBROMYALGIA

Maprotiline
BRAND NAMES: *Ludiomil*

DOSAGE: 25 to 150 mg per day in 1 to 3 doses

POSSIBLE SIDE EFFECTS: Blurred vision, decreased sexual ability, dizziness or lightheadedness, drowsiness, dry mouth, headache, increased or decreased sexual drive, tiredness or weakness

Trazodone
BRAND NAMES: *Desyrel, Trazon, Trialodine*

DOSAGE: 50 to 150 mg per day in 2 or 3 doses

POSSIBLE SIDE EFFECTS: Dizziness or lightheadedness, drowsiness, dry mouth, headache, nausea and vomiting, unpleasant taste in mouth

Drugs Used in Treating Arthritis

Zolpidem

BRAND NAMES: *Ambien*

DOSAGE: 10 mg per day in a single dose

POSSIBLE SIDE EFFECTS: Side effects are uncommon at prescribed dosage.

GOUT DRUGS

Allopurinol

BRAND NAMES: *Lopurin, Zyloprim*

DOSAGE: 100 to 300 mg per day in a single dose

POSSIBLE SIDE EFFECTS: Hives, itching, liver-function abnormalities, nausea, skin rash or sores

Colchicine

BRAND NAME: Available only as generic

DOSAGE: 0.6 to 1.2 mg per day in 1 to 2 doses for prevention. 0.5 or 0.6 mg every 1 or 2 hours (no more than 8 doses per day) to stop acute attacks.

POSSIBLE SIDE EFFECTS: Diarrhea, nausea and vomiting, stomach pain

Probenecid

BRAND NAMES: *Benemid, Probalan*

DOSAGE: 500 to 1,000 mg per day in 2 doses

POSSIBLE SIDE EFFECTS: Headache, joint pain and swelling, loss of appetite, nausea, skin rash, vomiting

Probenecid and colchicine

BRAND NAMES: *ColBenemid, Col-Probenecid, Proben-C*

DOSAGE: 1 tablet (500 mg probenecid and 0.5 mg colchicine) 1 or 2 times per day

POSSIBLE SIDE EFFECTS: Diarrhea, nausea and vomiting, stomach pain, headache, joint pain and swelling, loss of appetite, skin rash

Sulfinpyrazone

BRAND NAME: *Anturane*

DOSAGE: 100 to 800 mg per day in 1 or 2 doses

POSSIBLE SIDE EFFECTS: Lowered blood count, rash, stomach pain

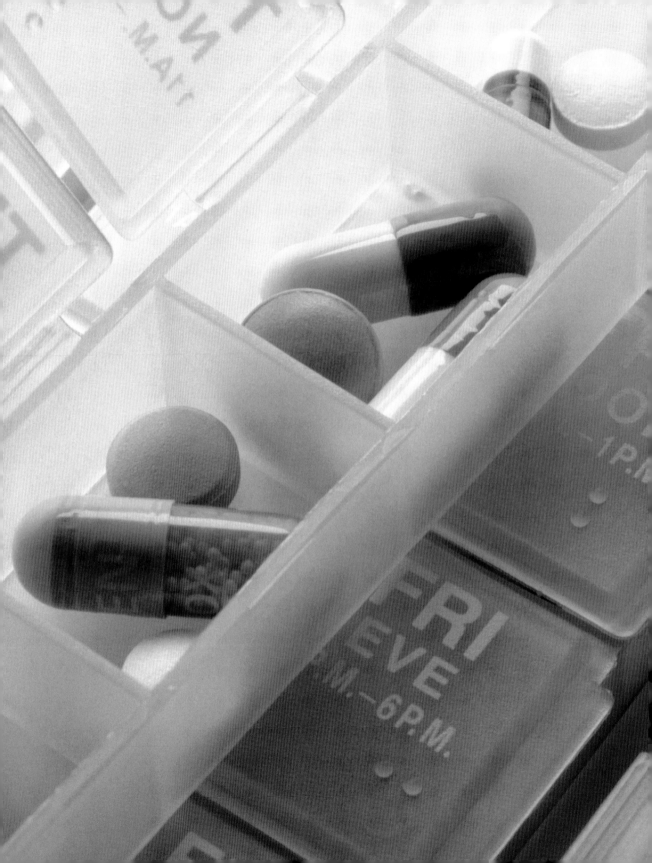

Combination Therapy
and Other Options

7

CHAPTER 7:
COMBINATION THERAPY AND OTHER OPTIONS

WHEN ONE DRUG ISN'T ENOUGH

Despite the plethora of medications available for treating almost every form of arthritis, it's unlikely that one drug will relieve all of your symptoms or that drugs alone will be the answer to treating your arthritis. Here, we will discuss what you can do when one drug isn't enough, and in later chapters, you'll learn about a variety of non-medication options that are equally important in managing your disease.

With all the drugs available, and new ones continuously being developed, there is some treatment to help almost anyone with arthritis. However, it's the rare individual who will find a single drug that works for all signs and symptoms of the disease. For most people, effectively treating arthritis requires a combination of drugs and other treatments.

For example, if you have rheumatoid arthritis, you may take an NSAID to help ease pain and inflammation and take a DMARD, or a combination of DMARDs, to get your disease under control. If you have lupus, you may take a DMARD, such as hydroxychloroquine sulfate (*Plaquenil*), to help control the disease, and a glucocorticoid medication to help prevent inflammation-related damage to internal organs such as the kidneys.

Not only will drugs most likely be used in combination with others, but the specific drugs and combinations can change over time, due to a number of factors, including the following situations.

When a Particular Drug No Longer Seems Effective

If you have been taking the same medication for your arthritis for a couple of years and notice that you're not doing as well as you were after your first months on the medication, it may be time to speak to your physician about trying a different medication or adding another drug.

Some drugs are highly effective when they are first prescribed, but seem to lose their effectiveness over time. It is not clear whether the drugs actually become less effective over time or whether the disease becomes more active. Regardless, a change in medication may be in order.

When You Need More Than One Drug

Just as different types of medications work to ease different signs and symptoms of disease, different DMARDs may be necessary, in some cases, to get the disease under control. If your old medication doesn't seem to be working as well as it used to, or if a DMARD hasn't produced the expected effects after a few months of use, your doctor may add a medication to the regimen, rather than switch to a new medication. The DMARD combinations used most commonly for RA include methotrexate (*Rheumatrex, Trexall*), hydroxychloroquine

(*Plaquenil*) and sulfasalazine (*Azulfidine, Azulfidine EN-Tabs*); and methotrexate and cyclosporine (*Neoral, Sandimmune*). Although research has shown such combinations are effective for some people, there have been no studies comparing the different DMARD combinations to one another.

Increasingly, doctors have begun to prescribe one of the new biologic agents with methotrexate for people with rheumatoid arthritis who do not achieve desired results with methotrexate alone. Some doctors also prescribe methotrexate with the new DMARD leflunomide (*Arava*).

Development of Other Medical Conditions

Some of the medications that help arthritis can actually worsen or cause unwanted effects in other diseases. For example, the development of hypertension might make it inadvisable to use glucocorticoid medications, which can contribute to high blood pressure. Kidney or liver disease may necessitate discontinuing certain gout medications or many disease-modifying drugs, such as azathioprine, cyclophosphamide and leflunomide, which are metabolized by the liver and excreted through the kidneys. Stomach ulcers may mean that you can't take certain NSAIDs or the osteoporosis drug alendronate, which can increase ulcer risk or worsen existing ulcers. Development of certain cancers or lupus-related blood clots, which estrogen can exacerbate, may mean you can't take estrogen replacement therapy for osteoporosis.

Even a natural condition like pregnancy can make a big difference in your medication regimen. While some arthritis medications are considered safe in pregnancy, several are off-limits, and the advisability of others depends on the particular stage of pregnancy.

Just as certain medical conditions may influence your doctor's prescribing decisions, so can the medications you take for those other conditions. In many cases, medications don't mix, so taking a certain medication for one condition may mean you have to forego a particular medication for another.

For example, if you have a clotting disorder that requires treatment with blood thinners, your doctor may advise against using aspirin and other NSAIDs that affect blood clotting. If you use antidepressant medications, your doctor may advise against your using narcotic analgesics for pain, because of the drugs' cumulative effects on the central nervous system. If you take allopurinol for gout, you may not be able to take the DMARD azathioprine (*Imuran*).

If the drugs you need to take for different conditions can't be taken together safely, your doctor will need to determine which of the drugs is more important for your health and well-being, and which drug is less essential or can be more safely or effectively replaced with another medication.

Nutritional supplements can have dangerous effects when mixed with prescription or over-the-counter medications. Nutritional supplements are products such as herbs, minerals and enzymes that are purported to promote good health but are not regulated by the FDA the way medications are. (For more on nutritional supplements, see Chapter 12, "Alternative

Therapies for Arthritis.") Several supplements, including the memory enhancer ginkgo biloba and the migraine remedy feverfew, can add to the blood-thinning effects of certain NSAIDs, possibly increasing a patient's risk of gastrointestinal bleeding.

In all cases, it's best to discuss with your doctor any medical problems you have, and the medications and nutritional supplements you take for them. Some health problems may make a difference in the medication you are prescribed initially, and some may necessitate changes in your current medication.

NEW TREATMENT APPROACHES

In addition to changes in or additions to medications, there are some new treatment approaches your doctor may use when the drugs you are taking don't control your disease. Here are some new options:

Viscosupplements

If you have OA pain of the knee that hasn't been relieved by NSAIDs or analgesic medications, or if you can't or choose not to take medications, a couple of relatively new products – hyaluronate sodium (*Hyalgan, Supartz*) and hylan G-F 20 (*Synvisc*) – may help.

Often referred to as viscosupplements, these products are delivered directly into the knee through a course of three or five injections. Although the products' action is not well understood, they are believed to work by replacing hyaluronic acid, a substance that gives joint fluid its viscosity. Hyaluronic acid production appears to break down in joints with OA.

Both products relieve pain and are most effective for people with mild to moderate knee OA. So far, the products are not approved for injection into joints other than the knee, nor is it known whether they would provide the same pain-relieving effects for other joints.

Prosorba Column Therapy

One of the newest approaches to the treatment of rheumatoid arthritis involves not medication, but a cylinder about the size of a soup can. The cylinder, called the *Prosorba* column, contains a sandlike substance, silica coated with protein A, which is a material that binds to antibodies associated with RA. The antibodies are then removed from the blood.

Protein A immunoadsorption therapy (*Prosorba* column therapy) is FDA-approved for people whose RA has not responded to disease-modifying antirheumatic drugs. The procedure typically takes place in a blood bank or a hospital's apheresis center. It is administered in 12 weekly sessions, each lasting two to two-and-a-half hours.

Exactly how the procedure reduces joint inflammation is unknown. Unwanted effects of treatment include a temporary, flu-like condition with chills, mild fever, nausea and fatigue. In rare cases, patients experience a rash that could make it necessary to discontinue treatment.

A TREATMENT FOR EVERYONE

By working closely with your physician and being open about how well a treatment is working or not working, you are almost certain to find a treatment or combination of treatments that will ease your symptoms and, perhaps, control your disease. The shortcoming of all arthritis medications, as well as the newer treatment options, however, is that none can undo the damage that arthritis already has caused.

Fortunately, in many cases, surgery can help. Through modern surgical techniques, orthopaedic surgeons can repair soft-tissue injuries and damage, and they can replace damaged joints with durable (and painless) synthetic ones.

Although most people with arthritis will never require joint replacement surgery, surgery of some type is fairly common in the treatment of joint injuries or arthritis.

In Chapter 8, we'll discuss some of the surgical options available when medications and other non-medication options aren't enough to manage the disease.

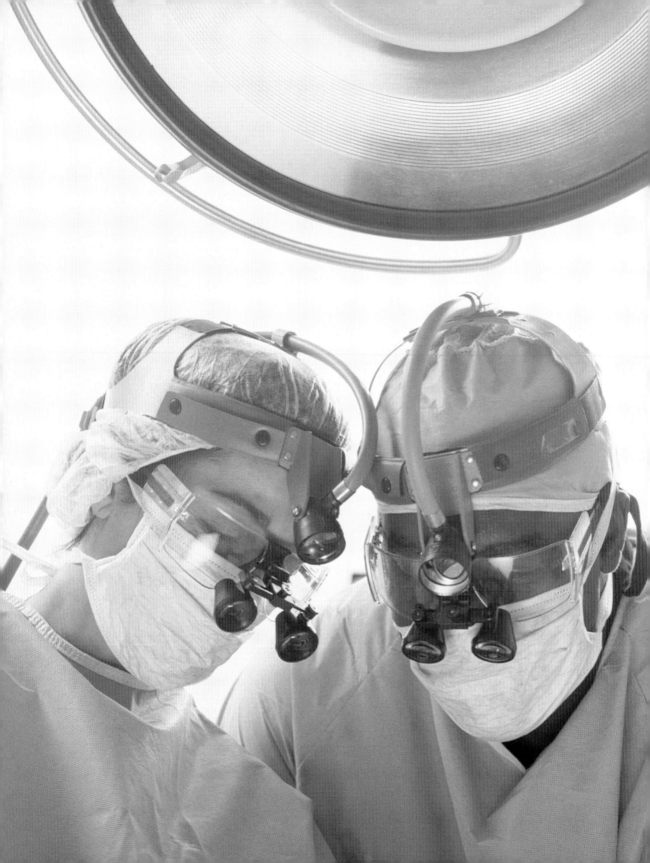

Surgery for Arthritis

8

CHAPTER 8: SURGERY FOR ARTHRITIS

For most people with arthritis, a combination of medications, exercise and joint protection techniques are sufficient for managing the disease. But when joint pain is severe and unrelenting, or when arthritis causes serious disability, surgery may be an effective option.

If you and your rheumatologist or primary-care physician believe that surgery is an appropriate option for you, your doctor will refer you to an orthopaedic surgeon, a doctor who specializes in surgery involving the musculoskeletal system. The surgeon can work with you to determine the type of surgery you need, how to prepare for surgery and what to expect before and after surgery. There are many different types of arthritis surgeries. The best type for you, should you need surgery, will depend on a number of factors, including the particular problem and its severity, the particular joint or joints involved, your age and your treatment goals.

DIFFERENT TYPES OF SURGERY

Surgery for arthritis is common, and the range of surgeries performed varies greatly – from simple outpatient procedures in which your joint damage is viewed through an arthroscope, to complete replacement of a damaged joint with a new prosthetic one.

Some surgeries may have you back to work within days, while others require months of activity limitations and physical therapy. What most of these surgeries have in common is that they offer the opportunity for less pain and improved function.

Here are some of the most common types of surgery for arthritis:

Synovectomy

Synovectomy is the removal of the diseased synovium or the membrane that lines the joint. In diseases like RA, the synovium becomes inflamed, causing joint pain, swelling and disability. Removing the synovium can reduce symptoms and prevent or slow destruction of the affected joint.

In most cases, a technique called synovectomy is performed through arthroscopy (see page 96). In some cases, particularly if a large joint is involved, a surgeon may use a large incision.

Synovectomy isn't always permanent. In time, the diseased synovium often grows back, necessitating another synovectomy or, possibly, joint replacement surgery.

Osteotomy

Osteotomy is the correction of bone deformity by cutting and repositioning the bone, then resetting it in a better position. The most common arthritis-related use of osteotomy for arthritis is to correct curving of the tibia (shin bone) and improve the weight-bearing position of the lower leg in people with osteoarthritis of the knee. Osteotomy of the pelvis may be used to correct misalignment of the hip joint that leads to excessive cartilage wear and damage, but in general, the predictability of success in osteotomy is less than that of total joint replacement. For some people, however, the procedure offers pain relief. Recovery and new bone growth take several weeks.

Resection

Resection involves removing a portion of the bone from a stiff or immobile joint, which creates a space between the bone and the joint. Although the bone itself never grows back, more flexible scar tissue fills the space and offers more flexibility. However, the joint is less stable. Resection is most common in upper extremities, such as the wrist, thumb or elbow, and in the foot.

Arthrodesis

Arthrodesis, also called bone fusion, relieves pain, usually in joints of the ankles, wrists, fingers and thumbs. In arthrodesis, the cartilage is removed from the ends of the two bones forming a joint, and the bones are positioned together and immobilized, often with a pin or rod. After a while, the two bones join to form a single, rigid unit. Although the fused joint loses flexibility, it can bear weight better, is more stable and no longer causes pain. In other words, the joint will be painless and sturdy, but you will not be able to bend it.

Arthrodesis often is used for joints that aren't commonly replaced with prostheses. It is effective for people who, for reasons such as joint infections or poor bone quality, aren't good candidates for total joint replacement surgery.

Arthroplasty or Total Joint Replacement

Arthroplasty, or total joint replacement, refers to the procedure by which damaged joints are surgically removed and replaced with metal, ceramic and plastic parts. This common procedure has been used widely for many years, with excellent results.

The joints replaced most commonly and successfully are those of the hip and knee. In fact, an estimated 179,000 knees and 125,000 hips are replaced in the United States each year. Smaller joints, including the shoulders, elbows and knuckles, also can be replaced.

When joint replacement was first performed in the 1960s, the prosthetic components were always cemented in place. The cement often cracked or broke down, causing the joint to loosen over the course of several years. Doctors began searching for a better way, and the search led to development of a new method called biologic fixation; to keep prosthetic joints in place, the surfaces of the prostheses are porous, allowing the patient's own bone to grow into the prosthesis and hold it in place.

For younger people who have good bone growth into the prosthesis, some doctors believe the result of an uncemented prosthesis may be a more durable, longer-lasting joint replacement. For older people, whose bone may not grow well enough to hold the prosthesis, cemented prostheses still are preferred. Sometimes, doctors use a hybrid joint, in which one component is cemented and the other is not. Fortunately, the development of better cements has improved the longevity of cemented joints. Because of this improvement, some doctors prefer to use cemented joints.

Whatever type of prosthesis is used, you can expect your new joint to last 10 to 15 years or

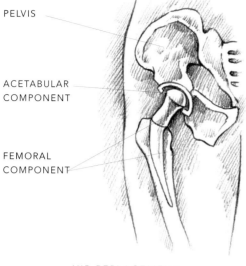

PELVIS

ACETABULAR
COMPONENT

FEMORAL
COMPONENT

HIP REPLACEMENT

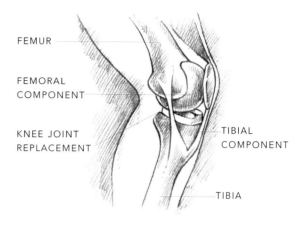

FEMUR

FEMORAL
COMPONENT

KNEE JOINT
REPLACEMENT

TIBIAL
COMPONENT

TIBIA

KNEE REPLACEMENT

more. If a joint wears out or loosens, a second joint surgery will be necessary to put in a new joint. Unfortunately, subsequent replacements tend to be less successful than initial ones, so doctors often prefer to postpone joint replacement for younger patients and reserve it for patients whose own life expectancy is closer to that of the prosthetic joints.

Arthroscopy

Arthroscopy is a process that allows a doctor to see directly into the joint through an arthroscope, a thin tube with a light at the end. An image of the joint's interior is transmitted to a closed-circuit television screen. The arthroscope is inserted through a small incision in the skin, and additional incisions may be used to insert small surgical tools.

Although you have probably heard about arthroscopy most often in connection with sports injuries in professional athletes, the procedure can be used for arthritis treatment and diagnostic purposes. Common uses for arthroscopy in treatment include removing a piece of loose tissue that is causing pain, repairing torn cartilage or smoothing a joint where the surface has become rough. More extensive surgery, such as synovectomy, or reconstruction of ligaments supporting a joint also can be done arthroscopically.

The advantage of arthroscopic surgery is that it requires less anesthesia and less cutting than a standard operation. It often is done on an outpatient basis, eliminating the need for a hospital stay. Furthermore, patients recover from arthroscopy much more quickly than they do from some other types of surgery, and they can get back to normal activities more quickly.

Arthroscopy is used most often on the knee or shoulder, but increasingly, it is being used to treat damage found in other joints affected by injury or arthritis, such as the elbow, hip, wrist and ankle.

IS SURGERY THE RIGHT OPTION?

If arthritis is disabling and hasn't responded to medical therapies or such non-medication treatments as physical therapy or exercise, or if you can't tolerate medications, surgery may be an appropriate option.

Your doctor and a surgeon will determine if surgery – and if, so what type of surgery – might help you. You will play a role in that decision, too, because in many cases, the decision to have surgery is a personal judgment call. Are you willing to undergo major surgery and weeks or months of rehabilitation for the prospect of having a pain-free joint and improved function, possibly for the rest of your life? Would you undergo the risks of surgery, such as potential infections, blood clots or anesthesia complications, for the opportunity to be mobile and maintain your independence?

As you consider whether or not to have surgery, keep in mind that every person's situation is different. You may not benefit from the same surgery that a friend, family member or the majority of participants in a medical study did. Your doctor may advise against a particular surgery or warn you that its chances of success are low. Even if your doctor thinks that surgery can help you, there are many factors that both you and your doctor must consider, including the following:

- **Other health problems.** If you have heart disease or lung disease, the strain of some types of surgery may be too much for you. Before having any kind of surgery, it's important to have other health problems under control.

- **Your medications.** In some cases, you may need to stop some of the medications you are taking for a while before surgery. For example, such drugs as aspirin and other nonsteroidal anti-inflammatory drugs, which you may be taking to ease pain and inflammation, may interfere with blood clotting and cause you to bleed excessively during surgery. On the other hand, glucocorticoid medications, such as prednisone, may be needed at larger doses during surgery. The reason is that these drugs are similar to hormones our bodies naturally produce in response to stress. In people who take synthetic glucocorticoids, the body's ability to increase its own production of these hormones may be hampered. Therefore, additional medication may be necessary to help your body meet the demands of the situation.

- **Infections.** If you have any type of bacterial infection in your body, even an abscessed tooth, you'll need to have it cleared up before you undergo any surgery. One possible problem after joint surgery is infection, which can spread from another part of your body to your joint through the bloodstream.

- **Your weight.** If you are overweight, it's best to start losing pounds before you decide to have surgery. Being overweight may put extra stress on your heart and lungs during surgery. If you are undergoing knee- or hip-replacement surgery, excess weight can be stressful on a prosthetic joint component. For any surgery involving a weight-bearing joint, excess body weight can make rehabilitation more difficult by placing strain on the joint and making it more difficult to do the exercises needed to make the joint stronger after surgery.

A modest loss of 10 percent of your body weight can make a difference, but for many people, losing such a small amount of weight takes a well-designed diet and exercise program as well as commitment and willpower. Consult your physician if you're not sure if you need to lose weight or, if you do need to lose, how to best go about it.

- **Strength and fitness.** Although any rehabilitation program after surgery will involve exercises to strengthen the muscles around the affected joint, doing such exercises beforehand may increase your odds of surgical success. Similarly, aerobic exercise can prepare your heart and lungs for the rigors of surgery and rehabilitation. To learn more about what you can do to improve your physical fitness before surgery, consult your doctor or a physical therapist.

- **Your care as you recuperate.** One of your major concerns as you consider surgery may be caring for yourself in the days and weeks that follow. Things to consider include: Who will care for your home, children, pets or plants while you are in the hospital? Who will care for you once you are home? Depending on the type of surgery you have, it may be a few days or a couple of months before you are able to do such things as stand for prolonged periods, drive a car, vacuum or shower without the assistance of another adult. Consider your personal support systems – or the possibility of hiring someone to help you for a while – before you schedule surgery.

If you properly prepare for surgery, you'll have less to do or be concerned about when the time arrives, and relieving yourself of that stress now may help you recuperate faster. Nevertheless, recovering from surgery – particularly major surgery, such as total joint replacement or resection – requires a commitment. The amount of work you put into a recovery process often makes the difference between success and failure and your risk of adverse effects. In general, here's what you can expect to do following major joint surgery.

- **Wear support hose.** Immediately after surgery and until you are up and moving, your doctor will have you wear tight, elastic hose, referred to as TED hose, on lower legs to prevent blood clots from forming in them. Blood clots, which can break loose and clog an artery, are among the most common and dangerous complications of joint replacement surgery.

- **Work your muscles.** Following surgery, and maybe even before, your doctor likely will refer you to a physical therapist who will give you a program of exercises that help strengthen the muscles that support the joint. It's important that you follow the program faithfully, even when it may be painful to do so, to gain as much use of the joint as possible.

Exercise will begin gradually and become progressively more strenuous as your joint gains strength and mobility.

- **Protect your joints.** Immediately after replacement surgery of the knee or hip, and for about six weeks after surgery, you'll need support when you walk. At first, you'll use a walker, and later, you'll graduate to a cane. You may need to wear a brace on the joint and use special, strategically placed pillows when you lie down.

Protecting a joint after surgery is important, regardless of the type of surgery you have. Your doctor, surgeon, nurse and physical therapist will give you advice on joint protection.

- **Heed limits.** As you start to feel better, you may be tempted to do too much too soon. Resist this temptation. Using your joint more than it's ready to be used, or moving the joint beyond its intended range of motion can cause damage and possibly necessitate further surgery. While prescribed exercise is essential, attempting to climb stairs, ride a horse or do jumping jacks shortly after joint replacement may cause your new joint to dislocate and can send you back to the hospital. If your new joint is one that relies on biologic fixation ("cementless" joint replacement) to stay in place, you may have more severe activity restrictions as the new bone grows into the prosthesis to hold it in place. Because joint cement hardens quickly, there may be fewer initial restrictions on a joint that is cemented in place.

Be sure to do all the exercises your doctor and physical therapist recommend, but also be sure to know and heed your joint's limits. If you have any doubt as to whether an activity is safe, consult your doctor.

- **Take your medications.** It's important that you take any medications your doctor prescribes exactly as directed. Medications you may need following surgery include narcotic analgesics to relieve pain and make it easier to perform your exercises; blood thinners to reduce the risk of blood clots; antibiotics to reduce infection risk; and, of course, any medications you need for your arthritis control, including any NSAIDs, glucocorticoids or DMARDs that you usually take. Although the joint on which you had surgery soon will feel better, unfortunately, the surgery will not slow damage or inflammation to other joints.

- **Steer clear of infection.** Even after you've recovered from surgery, it's important that you take extra precautions against bacterial infection if you have a joint prosthesis (or any type of implant in your body). For example, if you cut your finger on a kitchen knife or step on a nail, it's important that you ask your doctor about a course of antibiotics. Even something as seemingly innocuous as a dental cleaning or filling can introduce bacteria into the bloodstream. If you have a joint prosthesis, be sure to let your dentist know. He or she may want to prescribe antibiotics before working on your mouth. Any infection that enters the body through the bloodstream may settle in the joint, causing problems that can require further surgery to correct.

By properly preparing for joint surgery and following doctors' orders and common sense afterwards, your surgery may offer a lifetime of pain relief and increased mobility. As with any surgery, however, joint surgery offers no guarantees. In rare instances, joint surgery results in infection, which requires further treatment or surgery. Prostheses have a limited life expectancy in even the best of circumstances, so if you have joint replacement as a young adult or in middle age, there's a chance that the prosthesis will loosen and have to be replaced in time.

Because surgery may be less successful the second, or third, time around, and most people don't want to face the prospect of another surgery, age may be a major factor in your decision to have a joint replaced. Fortunately, there are many medications and other measures that can delay or eliminate the need for joint surgery. For those who do undergo joint replacement, advances in materials and surgical techniques are making the procedure work better and the joints last longer.

ANESTHESIA: TO SLEEP OR NOT TO SLEEP

Regardless of the type of surgery you have, it's almost a certainty that you will need some type of anesthesia. While most people associate anesthesia only with pain relief, it has an additional purpose in the operating room – it allows your surgeon and his team to control a wide range of natural bodily reflexes, such as heart rate and blood pressure, that could fluctuate dangerously in response to the trauma of surgery.

Your doctor will recommend one of three types of anesthesia – general, regional or local – to block your pain and control your natural bodily reflexes.

General Anesthesia

General anesthesia temporarily stops the brain's overall ability to sense and remember pain. Under general anesthesia, which you breathe in through a face mask, you are asleep. When you awaken, you may have vivid memories of the hours and minutes leading up to surgery. You may even remember being wheeled into the operating room and being asked to count backwards as the anesthetic put you to sleep. However, you will have no recollection of the time you are asleep or of the surgery itself.

Local or Regional Anesthesia

With both local and regional anesthesia, you are fully aware of what is going on during surgery and will remember the surgery. With local anesthesia, the doctor blocks the pain signal where the nerve begins. For a minor surgery of the foot, for example, he might administer a few localized injections that would numb just the foot.

For more complex knee surgery, on the other hand, your doctor might block pain responses from entire lower regions of the body by injecting an anesthetic into the outer covering of the spinal column (called *epidural anesthesia*).

With epidural anesthesia, you have full feeling in your upper body and will be able to speak with the surgical staff during the actual procedure.

Which Anesthesia Is Best?

The best anesthesia will depend on a number of factors, including your general health, the procedure you are having and personal preference. A local or regional anesthetic generally is less risky (see more about risks in Chapter 9), and you recover from it more quickly.

General anesthesia often is necessary for long, complicated surgeries. Even so, doctors often use regional anesthesia for such procedures as some joint replacement. Doing so may enable to you to be up and active more quickly, which may improve the odds of long-term success of the procedure.

QUESTIONS TO ASK YOUR DOCTOR ABOUT SURGERY

The decision to have surgery is a major one. You should collect as much information as possible about the surgery before you agree to it. Here are some questions you may want to ask your doctor and the surgeon to better understand the surgical procedure.

You also may find it helpful to talk to another person with your type of arthritis who has already had the surgery you are considering. (Your doctor may be able to refer you to another of his patients.) Some of these questions might be appropriate to ask that person, too. Remember: Every person and every surgery is different. Your surgery may not go exactly as another person's, even if your situations are similar.

- What other kinds of treatment could I have instead of surgery? How successful might those treatments be?
- Can you explain this surgical procedure, step by step?
- May I view materials or videos of this surgery?

- How long does this surgery typically take?
- Do you offer a class or informational meeting for people considering this surgery? (Some hospitals do.)
- May I have this surgery on an outpatient basis?
- What are the risks involved in the surgery? How likely are these risks?
- How can I avoid blood transfusions? What other options are there?
- What type of anesthesia will be used? What are the risks of anesthesia?
- How much improvement can I expect from the surgery?
- Will more surgery be necessary? After what period of time?
- If I choose to undergo this surgery, will you contact my family doctor? Will my primary-care physician be involved in my hospital stay? If so, in what way?
- Are you board-certified? Do you have a special interest or experience in arthritis surgery?
- What is your experience doing this type of surgery?
- Can you give me the name of someone

else who has undergone this surgery and who would talk to me about it?

- Is an exercise program recommended before and after the operation?
- Must I stop taking – or increase the dosage of – any of my medications before surgery?
- What happens if I delay surgery? Even for a few months?
- What are the risks if I don't have the surgery?

If you decide to proceed with surgery, here are some questions you will want to ask your doctor. You may wish to look over your insurance policy, if you have one, to be aware of your coverage for surgery.

- How long will I need to stay in the hospital after having the surgery?
- How much pain is involved? Will I receive medication for it? What kind of pain should I expect? How long will this pain last?
- How long do I have to stay in bed?
- When will I start physical therapy? Will I need home or outpatient therapy?

- Will in-hospital rehabilitation be covered by my insurance?
- May I review written material or videotapes about this phase of my care?
- Are physical therapy, occupational therapy and home health care covered by my insurance? For how long? (You may need to ask your insurance company about this and confirm what they will pay. Also, be aware that some insurance companies require a second opinion before authorizing any elective surgery.)
- Will I need to arrange for some assistance at home? If so, for how long?
- Will I need any special equipment for my home? Will I need to make any modifications to my home?
- What medications will I need for my recovery? How long will I need to take them?
- What limits will there be on my activities – driving, using the toilet, climbing stairs, bending, eating, having sex?
- How often will I have follow-up visits with you? Are they included in the cost of the surgery?

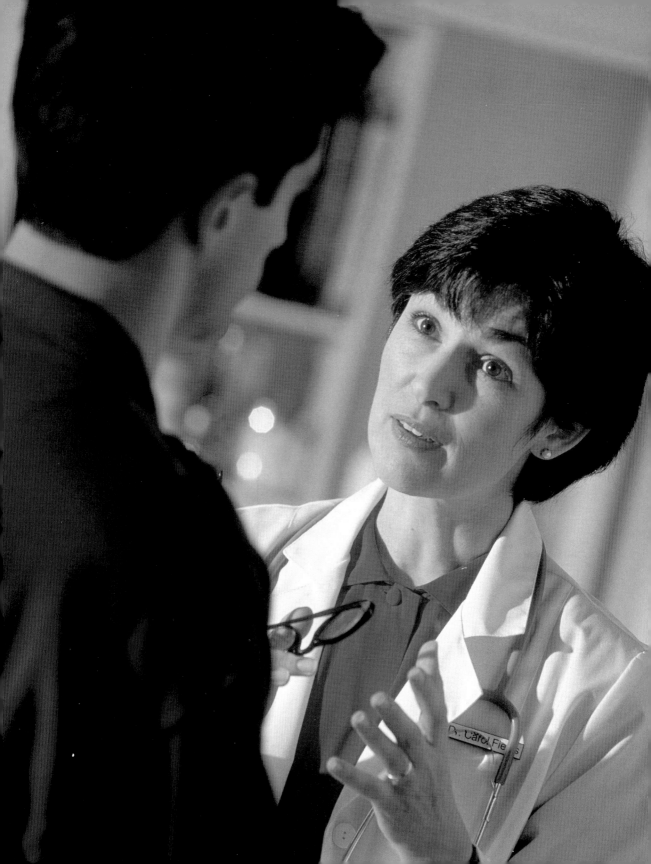

Complications and Side Effects

9

CHAPTER 9:
COMPLICATIONS AND SIDE EFFECTS

As with any medical treatment, there are benefits and drawbacks to arthritis treatment. Every medication or surgical procedure involves an element of risk. Making optimal treatment decisions for your particular condition requires understanding as much as you can about those risks as well as the potential benefits of the treatment.

Before doctors prescribe a medication or recommend a surgery, they consider what is called the risk/benefit ratio. That is, they estimate the risk of having the treatment and then compare that risk to the treatment's potential benefits. In other words, they weigh the potential risks of having a treatment against the risks of not having it. For example, if you had mild arthritis that caused only occasional pain and stiffness, your doctor would not be likely to prescribe a drug that causes severe side effects in even 10 percent of people who take it. In that case, the drug's potential risks clearly outweigh any benefits you might achieve from it.

On the other hand, if you have severe arthritis that is destroying your joints, or if you have a disease like lupus that is causing potentially life-threatening organ damage, even a certainty of some adverse effects might be preferable to not taking an otherwise helpful drug.

In most cases, the risk/benefit ratio is not so dramatic or clear-cut. In many cases, your doctor will rely largely on your judgment in the treatment process. After all, much of arthritis treatment involves judgment calls. Who can make those calls better than the person affected by them?

With some exceptions, treatment for most forms of arthritis is not a life-and-death matter. Rather, it's an issue of quality of life. Are you

MAKEOVER FOR MEDICATION LABELS

All nonprescription medications will soon will have a standard, easy-to-read label format, similar to the nutrition facts that started showing up on food products several years ago, that will help you better understand what you're buying. These labels, to be called "Drug Facts," will include such information as active ingredients, doses, warnings and a list of inactive ingredients, which can help consumers weed out products containing dyes or fillers to which they may be allergic.

The Food and Drug Administration, which has mandated the new labels, is requiring minimum type sizes and other graphic elements to ensure the labels' readability. By 2006, all over-the-counter medications should have the new labels.

DRUG RISKS

It's often said that anything strong enough to help is strong enough to harm. Any time you interfere with one bodily process to produce a desired effect, there's the chance that you'll produce a not-so-desirable effect somewhere else in the body. For example, a drug that suppresses your immune system so that it doesn't damage your joints may render your immune system less effective at fighting bacteria and viruses. The possible result: susceptibility to infection. A drug that suppresses inflammation-causing, hormone-like substances called prostaglandins may suppress similar substances that protect the stomach lining from digestive juices. The possible result: stomach ulcers and bleeding.

Almost every medication – even the so-called natural ones – is associated with some type of side effect. Many side effects resolve on their own, with time. Others require prompt attention by your physician. Still others are minor and may be necessary to live with if you are to receive the drugs' benefits.

If you experience any problems, no matter how minor, that you attribute to your medications, it's always best to speak with your physician. Depending on your reaction, your doctor may choose to adjust your dose, recommend measures to ease the side effects, switch you to another medication or advise you to bear with it.

For a listing of commonly used arthritis medications and side effects associated with them, see pages 73-85. Keep in mind that not all people taking these drugs will experience these side effects. But any potential side effect at least warrants a call to your doctor or pharmacist. With medications, conventional wisdom applies: Better safe than sorry.

willing to undergo the pain of surgery and a small risk of complications to be able to climb steps again or play on the floor with your grandchildren? Are you willing to put up with some medication-related nausea in return for the relief from progression of your arthritis that medication provides? Are you willing to undergo regular injections of medication and have regular blood tests to monitor the effects of a medication in order to lessen your chances of deformity or the need for surgery 10 years from now? These are the likely scenarios you'll be facing as you work with your doctor to determine your own risk/benefit ratio.

MINIMIZING YOUR RISK

Although some risk is inherent in any type of treatment you pursue, there are things you can do to minimize treatment risks, including the following:

Tell your doctor what medications you're taking. If your doctor prescribes a new medication, be sure to list all of the medications you are taking. If you are seeing more than one doctor for different medical conditions, it's possible that the doctor who treats your arthritis doesn't know about medications your other doctors have prescribed. Even if your doctor has noted such medications, it can't hurt to mention them again.

Let your doctor know if you are taking any over-the-counter medications, nutritional supplements or herbal remedies. Any of these agents has the potential to interact with or add to the effects of medications that your doctor prescribes. For example, if your doctor prescribes a nonsteroidal anti-inflammatory drug, such as ibuprofen or naproxen, and you already are taking an over-the-counter NSAID, such as *Advil, Motrin IB, Aleve or Orudis KT*, you could be setting yourself up for side effects, including gastric ulcers.

In some cases, a potential drug interaction may be reason enough for your doctor to prescribe a different drug for you. On the other hand, if potential benefits of the new drug (remember the risk/benefit ratio) are great enough to risk a potential reaction, the doctor may simply want to monitor you more closely so that any adverse effects can be caught early and, if necessary, one of the drugs can be discontinued.

Consider your lifestyle habits. If your doctor asks if you smoke or drink, answer truthfully.

If you aren't asked, offer the information. Lifestyle habits can make a difference in how medications work and can influence your risk of side effects. For example, drinking three or more drinks a day and taking acetaminophen could increase your risk of liver damage, and the same amount of alcohol could cause stomach bleeding in people taking NSAIDs. Since alcohol can increase the risk of liver damage from methotrexate therapy, most rheumatologists advise patients taking methotrexate to forego alcohol altogether or to limit their intake to only a small amount.

Consider your health risks. Health problems, such as kidney, liver or heart disease, ulcers, clotting disorders or cancer may influence your doctor's decision to recommend surgery or prescribe a particular medication. Many of these problems can be solved by prescribing a different medication or monitoring you carefully for the first signs of an adverse effect.

For example, a woman who has had breast cancer or who has a family history of breast cancer may not be able to take estrogen replacement hormone, the most common preventive treatment for osteoporosis. Estrogen has the potential to cause a worsening or recurrence of cancer. On the other hand, her doctor might prescribe one of the newer non-hormonal treatments for osteoporosis. Similarly, a person who has had ulcers probably wouldn't be a good candidate for traditional nonsteroidal anti-inflammatory drugs, which can increase ulcer risk. However, there are medications, such as nonacetylated salicylates or COX-2 inhibitors, that your doctor can pre-

AVOIDING MEDICAL MISTAKES

A person diagnosed with arthritis – or, in fact, just about any disease – has a rapidly expanding array of treatment options. Today's technology enables doctors to manage and treat disease better than at any time in history. Such advances are not without a price. Increasing numbers of medications and medical procedures – along with increasingly busy and rushed medical staffs trying to keep up with and administer them all – can lead to problems.

By being alert to problems that could occur and taking a role in your health care, you can reduce the chance of a potentially dangerous mistake. Here are some things you can do:

- Be sure you get the right drug. Because drugs designed for entirely different purposes can have names that sound alike, it's important that you make sure you are getting the right drug. If you have any doubt about what your doctor is prescribing, ask for the drug's name and its spelling (doctors' handwriting on prescription pads is notoriously hard to read). When you get your prescription filled, make sure you have the medication your doctor prescribed. Ask your pharmacist to confirm your prescription.

- Read medication labels. Always read and follow the directions on your prescription label. Problems can occur if you don't take a medication exactly as prescribed. Many pharmacies include a printed sheet with more extensive information about taking your drug. Read this sheet and ask your pharmacist or doctor any questions.

- Carefully reading – and heeding – labels on over-the-counter medications is essential. Fortunately, a recent FDA regulation is making over-the-counter medication labels easier to understand.

- Choose a high-volume hospital. If you are anticipating joint surgery, one of the best ways to increase the odds of its success is to find a surgeon and a hospital who perform many procedures of the particular surgery you will have.

- Take notes – or a friend. If you have difficulty remembering exactly what your doctor said once you leave the office, take notes. Another option is to take a friend or family member with you to your appointments. When it comes to comprehending and remembering important information, the old saying probably is right – two heads are better than one.

scribe to reduce pain and inflammation, and decrease ulcer risk.

Take your medication as prescribed. Adverse effects are more likely and a medication's benefits may be hampered if you don't take it exactly as prescribed. In general, it's best to take medications with a full glass of water. Be sure to ask your doctor or pharmacist about the best way to take your medication.

Some medications should be taken with food. Having a few crackers or a slice of bread, if not a full meal, can help reduce stomach upset associated with many drugs, but some drugs must be taken on an empty stomach to work. Others should not be taken with particular foods. If you have any doubts about how to take your medication, ask your physician or the pharmacist filling the prescription. It is always a good idea to read carefully any written material about your medications that the pharmacist provides.

Don't think that if one capsule helps a little, two or three ought to help a lot. Taking more than your prescribed dose of any medication can be dangerous.

If the medication you are taking is in liquid form, be sure to get a special measuring dropper or spoon to get the right dosage. The teaspoon you use for your morning cereal may be larger or smaller than an actual measuring spoon.

Let your doctor know if you experience any side effects. If you experience any problems that you attribute to a medication or you suspect that problems may be related to your medication, consult your doctor. The doctor may choose to change your medication dose, advise

you to wait out the problem or change the type of medicine.

Never stop taking a medication without first speaking to your doctor. If you're taking high

SURGERY RISKS & PREVENTION

Each year, joint replacement surgery gives almost half a million people the ability to move without pain for the first time in years, but it is not without risks. Here are some of the most common risks that you should be aware of before proceeding with joint surgery.

Blood clots. Joint surgery in general, and hip replacement in particular, carries the risk of blood-clot formation in the veins of the legs or the pelvis. While the clot is not dangerous in these areas, if it breaks loose and travels through the bloodstream to the lungs or another organ, it can cause organ damage, stroke or even death.

Prevention: With proper precautions, the risk of dangerous blood clots is slight. Preventive measures include the use of TED hose as prescribed by your physician, use of blood-thinning medications and getting out of bed and moving around as soon as advised by your physician. Clots are most likely to form in your body while you are lying still in bed.

Infection. There is the potential for infection with all surgical procedures. With total joint replacement, that risk exists not only at the doses of glucocorticoid medications, for example, or have been taking even a small dose over a long period of time, your doctor will need to wean you off of the medication. Stopping "cold turkey" can cause serious side effects, including a flare of the disease you are trying to control, fever, low blood pressure, or the inability to eat or even function.

time of surgery but afterwards, indefinitely. Any infection that enters the body through a cut or even a minor dental procedure has the potential to travel to and settle in the replaced joint.

Prevention: Antibiotics, usually given directly into the vein before and after surgery, can minimize the immediate risk. If you've had joint replacement surgery, you may need a preventative course of antibiotics before undergoing dental procedures.

Joint Dislocation.

When you have the ball-and-socket joint of the hip replaced, there is a slight risk that the ball of the prosthetic hip will slip out of the prosthetic socket. This risk is highest in the weeks just after surgery.

Prevention: To minimize the risk of a dislocation, it's important that you not bend your hip farther than a right (90-degree) angle. Twisting and crossing your legs also could put your new hip at risk. Speak to your physician about any particular exercises you should do or avoid to protect your hip.

Nerve Injury.

In extremely rare cases, the main nerve that supplies the leg may be damaged during hip replacement surgery. The result may be difficulty moving the foot up and down or feelings of pins and needles in the affected leg.

Prevention: Although there is nothing you can do to prevent nerve damage, in the rare event that this occurs, it helps to know that such damage usually heals on its own, restoring full movement and feeling to the leg.

Loosening.

Although loosening of the prosthesis is, perhaps, the most common risk of joint replacement, it usually doesn't occur until at least 10 years after you have had the surgery.

Prevention: Aside from improved surgical techniques and materials, there probably is no way to prevent loosening. However, it's important that you report any unusual pain around the replaced joint – particularly after the incision has healed – to your doctor. Pain can be a sign that the joint has loosened and further surgery is necessary to correct the problem. Because not all joint loosening is painful, doctors often order periodic X-rays following surgery to make sure that the new joint is firmly in place.

When you fill a prescription, the pharmacy likely will provide you with a sheet of information about how to take the drug and any side effects associated with the drug. Read over the sheet and become familiar with any potential side effects that warrant medical attention.

Follow doctor's orders. Just as you must follow a medication prescription precisely, it's important that you do as your doctor advises. (In fact, his advice concerning a medication should supersede what you see on the medication label.) If he says not to climb stairs for two weeks after surgery, for example, don't climb stairs three days later. You could be setting yourself up for problems.

Beware of medical errors. Many problems with arthritis treatment are not inherent with the treatment, but are the result of medical errors. Taking the wrong medication for your condition or having the wrong joint operated on are obvious examples of serious medical errors, but they are not the only ones. By using caution and taking an active role in your health care, you can help reduce your risk of errors. For more advice on protecting yourself, see "Avoiding Medical Mistakes" on page 109.

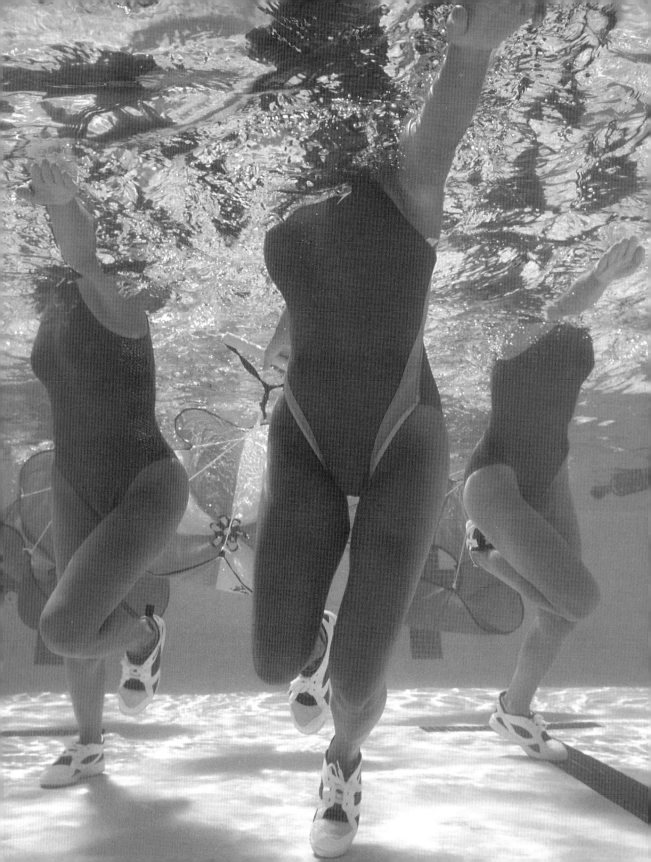

Other Ways to Ease Symptoms

10

CHAPTER 10:
OTHER WAYS TO EASE SYMPTOMS

Although arthritis medications (and in certain cases, surgery) can improve pain, reduce swelling, prevent or, in the case of surgery, correct, deformity, they are not the whole solution. Far from it. There are many other things your doctor or other health professional can do for you and, even more importantly, that you can do for yourself.

In this chapter, we'll discuss some of the many methods – beyond medication and surgery – you may find helpful in easing the pain, stiffness and other symptoms of arthritis. Some of these – such as using hot and cold – you can begin right now at home. For others, you'll need the help of a health-care professional. And, if you are considering significant changes in your diet or exercise level, it's always a good idea to first consult your physician.

EXERCISE

One of the best things you can do for yourself, whether or not you have arthritis, is to get regularly exercise. You don't have run a marathon or bench-press your body weight to see the benefits of exercise. Something as simple as walking, gardening, raking leaves, golfing or taking a water exercise class at your local community center can help ease pain, stiffness and joint mobility problems.

Regular exercise has a number of benefits for people with arthritis. It can help you:

- Keep your joints moving, which increases their range of motion and helps ease stiffness;
- Strengthen muscles that support the joint, lightening the stressful load that fragile joints must bear;
- Keep bones strong and healthy, which reduces your risk of osteoporosis;
- Help you perform your daily activities more easily and, perhaps, maintain your independence until late in life, despite arthritis;
- Maintain your weight or lose weight, which can lessen stress on weight-bearing joints such as the hip and knee;
- Increase your energy and improve your sleep, both of which can be affected adversely by a chronic, painful disease like arthritis;
- Ease pain, by prompting your body to produce its own natural painkillers called endorphins;
- Improve your self-esteem, by showing you that you can be strong and active, despite arthritis;
- Make you healthier, by reducing your risk of such problems as heart disease, lung disease and certain cancers.

A regular exercise program should consist of three types of exercise:
- Range-of-motion exercises, which keep your joints flexible, may involve bending, stretching or swaying.
- Isometric exercises, in which a force is applied to a resistant object. An example would

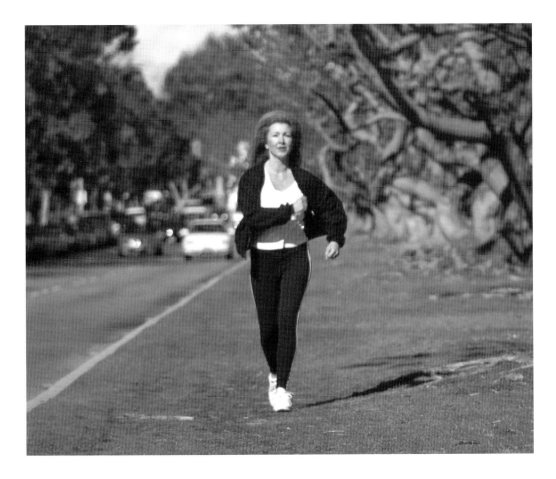

be placing both palms together, upright, in front of you (as if you are praying) and pressing them against each other. Isometric exercises can be helpful in strengthening muscles that support arthritic joints.

- Aerobic or endurance exercises, which involve sustained use of large muscles and increased heart rate, will strengthen your heart and lungs. Aerobic exercise includes dancing, fast walking, swimming and jogging.

If your arthritis involves your hips, knees or the joints of your feet, it's best to avoid jarring exercises, such as high-impact (or "regular") aerobics, running or jogging. For most people with arthritis, swimming, low-impact aerobics, walking, weightlifting, riding a stationary cycle or taking part in an aquatic exercise program (see Arthritis Foundation Aquatics Program on page 132) are safe and beneficial. The Arthritis Foundation offers a variety of exercise videos to help you get in shape and loosen joints. Information about these tapes is included in the Resources section at the end of this book.

Sample Exercises for Arthritis

Here are some sample exercises for general flexibility and strengthening that you can use to warm up or cool down. Try these exercises along with an aerobic exercise routine (such as walking or swimming) approved by your doctor. Note the precautions, if any, and choose the exercises that are best for you, depending on which areas of your body are painful. Always check with your doctor before beginning any new exercise program or routine, and describe what form of exercise you are considering. These suggested exercises are based on the Arthritis Foundation's PACE (People with Arthritis Can Exercise) program. For information, contact your local Arthritis Foundation chapter.

In addition to aerobic exercises such as walking, swimming or bicycling, many people with arthritis find benefit in gentle exercise alternatives, such as yoga, tai chi or *qi gong*. For some, the appeal of these alternatives is the ease and gentleness of the movements and the fact that they can be done in a small space with no special clothing or equipment. For others, these alternatives add variety to their exercise program. More information is on page 131.

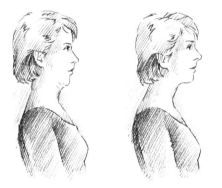

1. CHIN TUCKS
PULL YOUR CHIN BACK AS IF TO MAKE A DOUBLE CHIN. KEEP YOUR HEAD STRAIGHT – DON'T LOOK DOWN. HOLD THREE SECONDS. THEN RAISE YOUR NECK STRAIGHT UP AS IF SOMEONE WAS PULLING STRAIGHT UP ON YOUR HAIR.

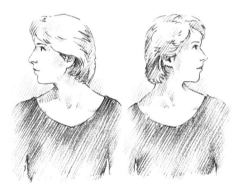

2. HEAD TURNS (ROTATION)
TURN YOUR HEAD TO LOOK OVER YOUR SHOULDER. HOLD THREE SECONDS. RETURN TO THE CENTER AND THEN TURN TO LOOK OVER YOUR OTHER SHOULDER. HOLD THREE SECONDS. REPEAT.

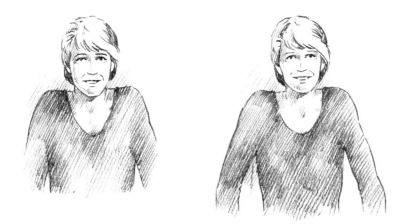

3. SHOULDER CIRCLES

LIFT BOTH SHOULDERS UP, MOVE THEM FORWARD, THEN DOWN AND BACK IN A CIRCLING MOTION. THEN LIFT BOTH SHOULDERS UP, MOVE THEM BACKWARD, THEN DOWN AND FORWARD IN A CIRCLING MOTION.

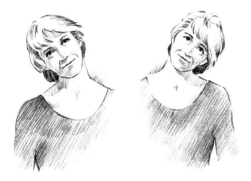

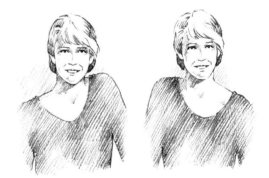

4. HEAD TILTS

FOCUS ON AN OBJECT IN FRONT OF YOU. TILT YOUR HEAD SIDEWAYS TOWARD YOUR RIGHT SHOULDER. HOLD THREE SECONDS. RETURN TO THE CENTER AND TILT TOWARD YOUR LEFT SHOULDER. HOLD THREE SEC-ONDS. DO NOT TWIST HEAD BUT CONTINUE TO LOOK FORWARD. DO NOT RAISE YOUR SHOULDER TOWARD YOUR EAR.

5. SHOULDER SHRUGS

(A) RAISE ONE SHOULDER, LOWER IT. THEN RAISE THE OTHER SHOULDER. BE SURE THE FIRST SHOULDER IS COMPLETELY RELAXED AND LOWERED BEFORE RAISING THE OTHER.
(B) RAISE BOTH SHOULDERS UP TOWARD THE EARS. HOLD THREE SECONDS. RELAX. CONCEN-TRATE ON COMPLETELY RELAXING SHOULDERS AS THEY COME DOWN. DO NOT TILT THE HEAD OR BODY IN EITHER DIRECTION. DO NOT HUNCH YOUR SHOULDERS FORWARD OR PINCH SHOUL-DER BLADES TOGETHER.

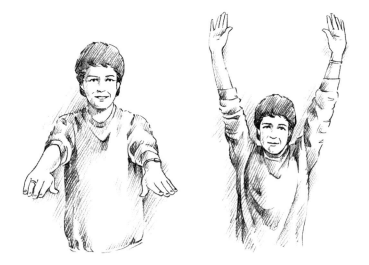

6. FORWARD ARM REACH

RAISE ONE OR BOTH ARMS FORWARD AND UPWARD AS HIGH AS POSSIBLE. RETURN TO YOUR
STARTING POSITION.

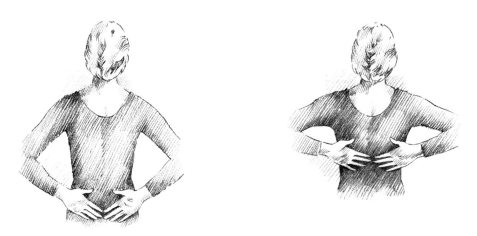

7. SELF BACK RUB

WHILE SEATED, SLIDE A FEW INCHES FORWARD FROM THE BACK OF YOUR CHAIR. SIT UP AS
STRAIGHT AS POSSIBLE; DO NOT ROUND YOUR SHOULDERS. PLACE THE BACK OF YOUR HANDS
ON YOUR LOWER BACK. SLOWLY MOVE THEM UPWARD UNTIL YOU FEEL A STRETCH IN YOUR
SHOULDERS. HOLD THREE SECONDS, THEN SLIDE YOUR HANDS BACK DOWN. YOU CAN USE ONE
HAND TO HELP THE OTHER. MOVE WITHIN THE LIMITS OF YOUR PAIN. DO NOT FORCE.

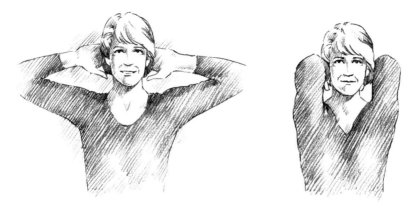

8. SHOULDER ROTATOR

SIT OR STAND AS STRAIGHT AS POSSIBLE. REACH UP AND PLACE YOUR HANDS ON THE BACK OF YOUR HEAD. (IF YOU CANNOT REACH YOUR HEAD, PLACE YOUR ARMS IN A "MUSCLE MAN" POSITION WITH ELBOWS BENT IN A RIGHT ANGLE AND UPPER ARM AT SHOULDER LEVEL.) TAKE A DEEP BREATH IN. AS YOU BREATHE OUT, BRING YOUR ELBOWS TOGETHER IN FRONT OF YOU. SLOWLY MOVE ELBOWS APART AS YOU BREATHE IN.

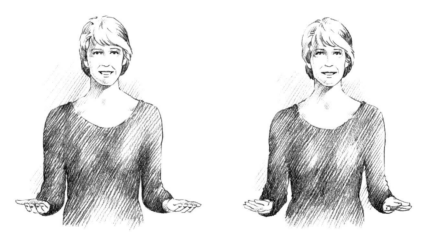

9. DOOR OPENER

BEND YOUR ELBOWS AND HOLD THEM IN TO YOUR SIDES. YOUR FOREARMS SHOULD BE PARALLEL TO THE FLOOR. SLOWLY TURN FOREARMS AND PALMS TO FACE THE CEILING. HOLD THREE SECONDS AND THEN TURN PALMS SLOWLY TOWARD THE FLOOR.

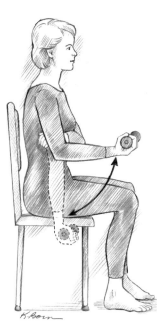

10. BICEPS CURL

SIT IN A CHAIR, FEET ON THE FLOOR. HOLD A ONE-POUND WEIGHT IN YOUR RIGHT HAND, LETTING YOUR ARM HANG AT YOUR SIDE. BRING YOUR LEFT ARM ACROSS YOUR CHEST, RESTING THE BACK OF YOUR RIGHT ARM ON YOUR LEFT FIST. SLOWLY BEND YOUR ELBOW, TURNING YOUR RIGHT FOREARM TOWARD THE FRONT OF YOUR SHOULDER. YOUR PALM SHOULD BE FACING YOUR SHOULDER. PAUSE, THEN LOWER YOUR ARM TO THE COUNT OF THREE. REPEAT ON THE LEFT SIDE.

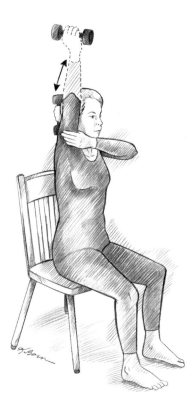

11. OVERHEAD TRICEPS

SIT IN A CHAIR, HOLDING A ONE-POUND WEIGHT IN YOUR RIGHT HAND. BRING YOUR RIGHT ARM ABOVE YOUR HEAD, STOPPING WHEN THE INSIDE OF YOUR ELBOW IS ABOVE YOUR RIGHT EAR. SUPPORT YOUR RIGHT UPPER ARM WITH YOUR LEFT HAND. SLOWLY BEND YOUR RIGHT ELBOW, LOWERING THE WEIGHT TO YOUR RIGHT SHOULDER. STRAIGHTEN YOUR ELBOW TO THE COUNT OF THREE, PAUSE, THEN LOWER IT BACK TO YOUR SHOULDER. REPEAT WITH THE LEFT ARM.

(THESE TWO EXERCISES ADAPTED FROM *ARTHRITIS TODAY*)

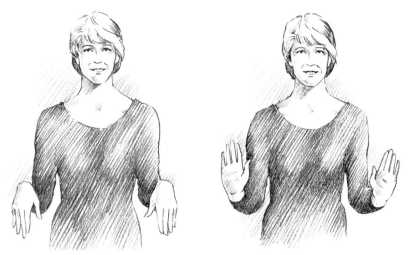

12. WRIST BEND

IF SITTING, REST HANDS AND FOREARMS ON THIGHS, TABLE, OR ARMS OF CHAIR. IF STANDING, BEND YOUR ELBOWS AND HOLD HANDS IN FRONT OF YOU, PALMS DOWN. LIFT PALMS AND FINGERS, KEEPING FOREARMS FLAT. HOLD THREE SECONDS. RELAX.

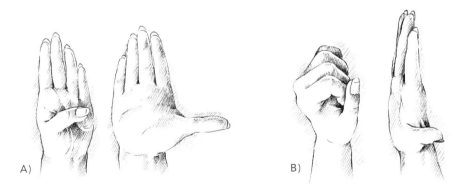

A)

B)

13. THUMB BEND AND FINGER CURL

(A) WITH HANDS OPEN AND FINGERS RELAXED, REACH THUMB ACROSS YOUR PALM AND TRY TO TOUCH THE BASE OF YOUR LITTLE FINGER. HOLD THREE SECONDS. STRETCH THUMB BACK OUT TO THE OTHER SIDE AS FAR AS POSSIBLE.

(B) MAKE A LOOSE FIST BY CURLING ALL YOUR FINGERS INTO YOUR PALM. KEEP YOUR THUMB OUT. HOLD FOR THREE SECONDS. THEN STRETCH YOUR FINGERS TO STRAIGHTEN THEM.

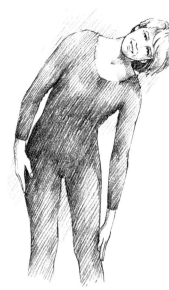

14. SIDE BENDS

WHILE STANDING, KEEP WEIGHT EVENLY ON BOTH HIPS WITH
KNEES SLIGHTLY BENT. LEAN TOWARD THE RIGHT AND REACH
YOUR FINGERS TOWARD THE FLOOR. HOLD THREE SECONDS.
RETURN TO CENTER AND REPEAT EXERCISE TOWARD THE LEFT.
DO NOT LEAN FORWARD OR BACKWARD WHILE BENDING,
AND DO NOT TWIST THE TORSO.

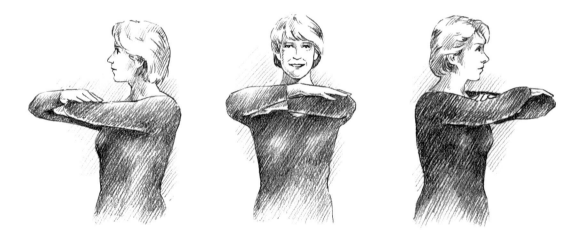

15. TRUNK TWIST

PLACE YOUR HANDS ON YOUR HIPS, STRAIGHT OUT TO THE SIDE, CROSSED OVER YOUR CHEST,
OR ON OPPOSITE ELBOWS. TWIST YOUR BODY AROUND TO LOOK OVER YOUR RIGHT SHOULDER.
HOLD THREE SECONDS. RETURN TO THE CENTER AND THEN TWIST TO THE LEFT. BE SURE YOU
ARE TWISTING AT THE WAIST AND NOT AT YOUR NECK OR HIPS. NOTE: VARY THE EXERCISE BY
HOLDING A BALL IN FRONT OF OR NEXT TO YOUR BODY.

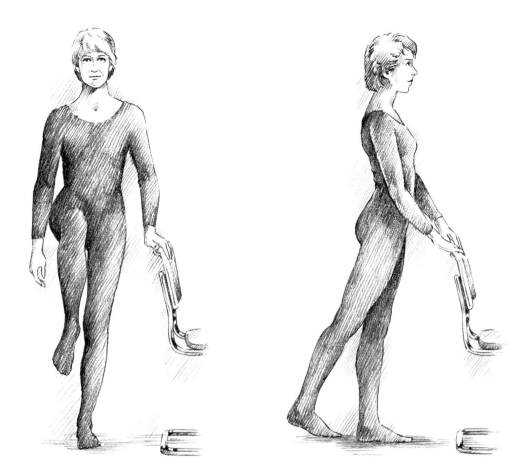

16. MARCH

STAND SIDEWAYS TO A CHAIR AND LIGHTLY GRASP THE BACK. IF YOU FEEL UNSTEADY, HOLD ONTO TWO CHAIRS OR FACE THE BACK OF THE CHAIR. ALTERNATE LIFTING YOUR LEGS UP AND DOWN AS IF MARCHING IN PLACE. GRADUALLY TRY TO LIFT KNEES HIGHER AND/OR MARCH FASTER.

17. BACK KICK

STAND STRAIGHT ON ONE LEG AND LIFT THE OTHER LEG BEHIND YOU. HOLD THREE SEC-ONDS. TRY TO KEEP YOUR LEG STRAIGHT AS YOU MOVE IT BACKWARD. MOTION SHOULD OCCUR ONLY IN THE HIP (NOT THE WAIST). DO NOT LEAN FORWARD – KEEP YOUR UPPER BODY STRAIGHT. NOTE: YOU CAN ADD RESIS-TANCE BY USING A LARGE RUBBER EXERCISE BAND AROUND ANKLES.

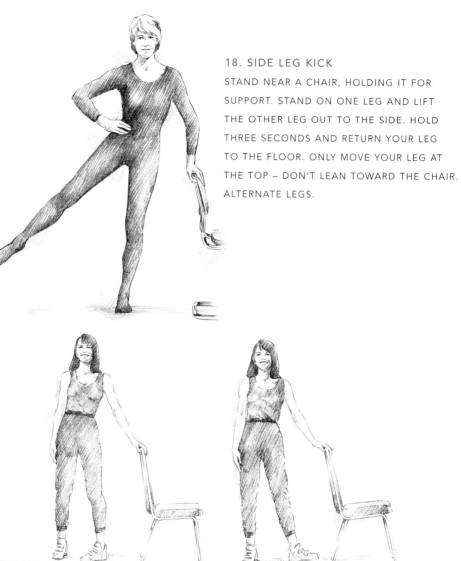

18. SIDE LEG KICK

STAND NEAR A CHAIR, HOLDING IT FOR SUPPORT. STAND ON ONE LEG AND LIFT THE OTHER LEG OUT TO THE SIDE. HOLD THREE SECONDS AND RETURN YOUR LEG TO THE FLOOR. ONLY MOVE YOUR LEG AT THE TOP – DON'T LEAN TOWARD THE CHAIR. ALTERNATE LEGS.

19. HIP TURNS

STAND WITH LEGS SLIGHTLY APART, WITH YOUR WEIGHT ON ONE LEG AND THE HEEL OF YOUR OTHER FOOT LIGHTLY TOUCHING THE FLOOR. ROTATE YOUR WHOLE LEG FROM THE HIP SO THAT TOES AND KNEE POINT IN AND THEN OUT. DON'T ROTATE YOUR BODY – KEEP CHEST AND SHOULDERS FACING FORWARD. NOTE: IF YOU HAVE DIFFICULTY PUTTING WEIGHT ON ONE LEG, YOU CAN DO THIS EXERCISE BY SITTING AT THE EDGE OF A CHAIR WITH YOUR LEGS EXTENDED STRAIGHT IN FRONT AND YOUR HEELS RESTING ON THE FLOOR.

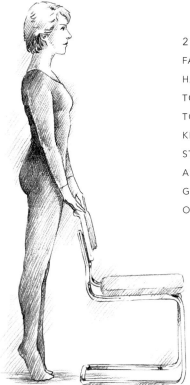

21. TIPTOE

FACE THE BACK OF A CHAIR AND REST YOUR HANDS ON IT. RISE AND STAND ON YOUR TOES. HOLD THREE SECONDS, THEN RETURN TO THE FLAT POSITION. TRY TO KEEP YOUR KNEES STRAIGHT (BUT NOT LOCKED). NOW STAND ON YOUR HEELS, RAISING YOUR TOES AND FRONT PART OF YOUR FOOT OFF THE GROUND. NOTE: YOU CAN DO THIS EXERCISE ONE FOOT AT A TIME.

20. SKIER'S SQUAT
(QUADRICEPS STRENGTHENER)

STAND BEHIND A CHAIR WITH YOUR HANDS LIGHTLY RESTING ON TOP OF THE CHAIR FOR SUPPORT. KEEP YOUR FEET FLAT ON THE FLOOR. KEEPING YOUR BACK STRAIGHT, SLOWLY BEND YOUR KNEES TO LOWER YOUR BODY A FEW INCHES. HOLD FOR THREE TO SIX SECONDS, THEN SLOWLY RETURN TO AN UPRIGHT POSITION.

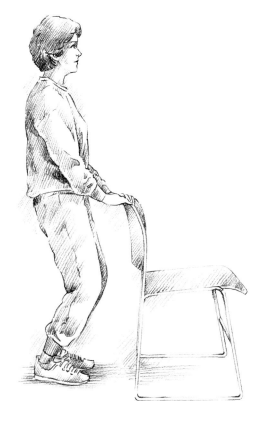

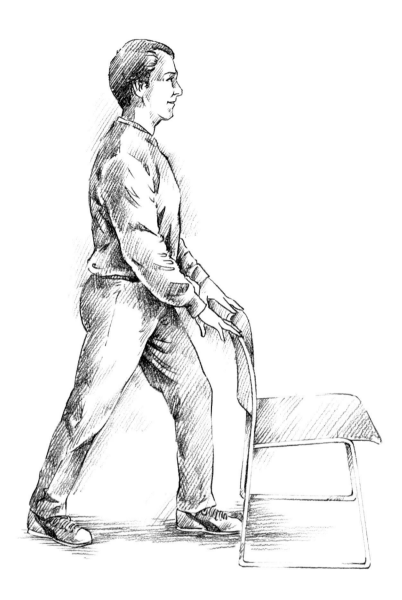

22. CALF STRETCH

HOLD LIGHTLY TO THE BACK OF A CHAIR. BEND THE KNEE OF THE LEG YOU ARE NOT STRETCHING
SO THAT IT ALMOST TOUCHES THE CHAIR. PUT THE LEG TO BE STRETCHED BEHIND YOU, KEEPING
BOTH FEET FLAT ON THE FLOOR. LEAN FORWARD GENTLY, KEEPING YOUR BACK KNEE STRAIGHT.

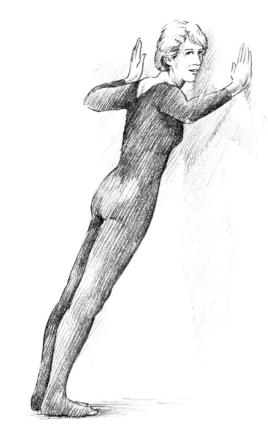

23. CHEST STRETCH

STAND ABOUT TWO TO THREE FEET AWAY FROM A WALL AND PLACE YOUR HANDS OR FOREARMS ON THE WALL AT SHOULDER HEIGHT. LEAN FORWARD, LEADING WITH YOUR HIPS. KEEP YOUR KNEES STRAIGHT AND YOUR HEAD BACK. HOLD THIS POSITION FOR FIVE TO 10 SECONDS, THEN PUSH BACK TO STARTING POSITION. TO FEEL MORE STRETCH, PLACE YOUR HANDS FARTHER APART.

24. THIGH FIRMER AND KNEE STRETCH

SIT ON THE EDGE OF YOUR CHAIR OR LIE ON YOUR BACK WITH YOUR LEGS STRETCHED OUT IN FRONT AND YOUR HEELS RESTING ON THE FLOOR. TIGHTEN THE MUSCLE THAT RUNS ACROSS THE FRONT OF THE KNEE BY PULLING YOUR TOES TOWARD YOUR HEAD. PUSH THE BACK OF THE KNEE DOWN TOWARD THE FLOOR SO YOU ALSO FEEL A STRETCH AT THE BACK OF YOUR KNEE AND ANKLE. FOR A GREATER STRETCH, PUT YOUR HEEL ON A FOOTSTOOL AND LEAN FORWARD AS YOU PULL YOUR TOES TOWARD YOUR HEAD.

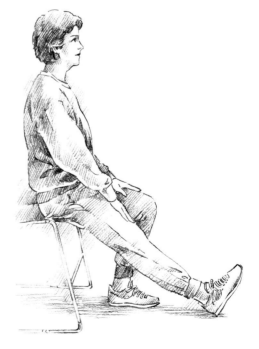

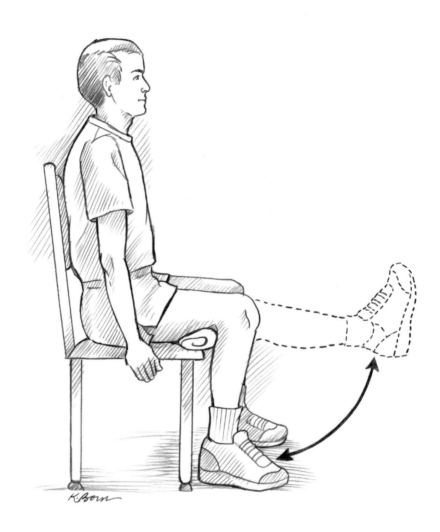

K. Born

25. KNEE EXTENSION

SIT IN A CHAIR WITH YOUR FEET SHOULDER-WIDTH APART, KNEES DIRECTLY ABOVE THEM. PUT A TOWEL UNDER YOUR KNEES FOR PADDING. WITH YOUR HANDS ON YOUR THIGHS, RAISE YOUR RIGHT LEG TO THE COUNT OF THREE UNTIL YOUR KNEE IS STRAIGHT (BUT NOT LOCKED). PAUSE, THEN LOWER YOUR LEG TO THE COUNT OF THREE. REPEAT ON THE LEFT SIDE.

(THIS EXERCISE ADAPTED FROM *ARTHRITIS TODAY*.)

Yoga

Practiced around the world, yoga is part of the traditional Indian healing system called Ayurveda. Although there are several branches of yoga practice, the form you're most likely familiar with is hatha yoga. Hatha yoga consists of balancing exercises and gentle stretches that condition the whole body.

Practicing yoga daily can improve flexibility and balance and increase muscles. It also can help you relax. If you are interested in trying yoga, many colleges, community centers, senior centers, health clubs and even workplaces offer yoga classes.

Before signing up for a yoga class, it's best to speak with your physician. Some types of yoga are more strenuous than others. You need to find an instructor who is familiar with arthritis and who will be sensitive to your limitations if there are moves that you can't do comfortably. Once you have learned yoga from a competent instructor, you may want to practice with an instructional videotape. Your doctor, yoga instructor or physical therapist may be able to recommend a good videotape that is appropriate for people with arthritis.

Tai chi

Although its roots are in martial arts, tai chi is not confrontational. It consists of controlled movements that flow rhythmically into one long, graceful gesture. Research has shown that tai chi improves balance and reduces the risk of falling, which could be serious for a person with fragile bones and joints. At least one study has suggested that tai chi is safe for people with rheuma-toid arthritis. Because of its gentle, graceful movements, it's a popular form of exercise for people with many different forms of arthritis. There are many more videos and books, along with community classes, providing instruction in tai chi. Consult your health-care professional.

Qi Gong

Qi gong (pronounced chee kung) has been practiced in Asia for more than 3,000 years to promote health and self-healing. There are several styles of qi gong, which involve meditation, breathing exercises and movements. In general, qi gong is less graceful than tai chi, and some styles are more active than others. Qi gong exercises can be practiced by people of all ages and fitness levels. They can even be done from a bed or wheelchair.

Although the qi gong has not been well-studied for arthritis, in a 1998 study of fibromyalgia patients, those using qi gong with meditation reported improvement in depression, coping skills, pain and function.

If you have any questions about a particular exercise or would like an exercise program suited to your particular condition and needs, consult a physical therapist.

PHYSICAL THERAPY

Despite the proven and varied benefits of exercise, if you have arthritis, you should not begin an exercise program without consulting your doctor – particularly if your arthritis has caused you to be sedentary for some time. Your doctor may want to give you a physical evaluation or refer you to a physical therapist.

ARTHRITIS FOUNDATION AQUATICS PROGRAM

The Arthritis Foundation Aquatics Program (AFAP) is a water exercise program designed for people with arthritis and related conditions. Classes usually are conducted two to three times per week at local indoor pools for 45 to 60 minutes. Instructors have completed an Arthritis Foundation-approved training program. Although AFAP will not replace the exercises prescribed by your doctor or physical therapist, participants do report such physical benefits as decreased pain and stiffness after taking part in the classes.

Joining a water exercise class gives you the opportunity to exercise in warm water, with guidance from a trained instructor. It also gives you the opportunity to socialize regularly with other people who have conditions similar to yours. For more information about AFAP, contact your local office of the Arthritis Foundation. To find the Arthritis Foundation office that serves your area, call 800/283-7800 or visit the Arthritis Foundation Web site at www.arthritis.org.

A physical therapist (PT) is a health-care professional who helps people with arthritis by teaching them to do exercises designed to meet certain goals. Unlike a personal trainer, whose goal may be to help you firm your thighs and look better in a bathing suit, a physical therapist's goal is to help you function better.

The college coursework required to complete a physical therapy degree includes basic science courses, such as biology, chemistry and physics, and more specialized courses, such as biomechanics, manifestations of disease, examination techniques and therapeutic procedures. To practice, degreed physical therapists must pass a licensure exam in their state.

Physical therapy generally begins with a complete assessment of the joints to determine range of motion and muscle strength. The physical therapist may ask to see you walk and question you about any joints that are painful.

Once the assessment is complete, the therapist will prescribe a program of exercise to improve your joints' range of motion and increase the strength of muscles supporting arthritic joints. He or she may recommend a program of aerobic exercise that will not damage your joints, and may prescribe devices to help address any particular problems you are having. These devices could include a crutch or cane to help you walk with an arthritic knee, or a shoe insert to ease painful feet or compensate for a discrepancy in leg length, which may contribute to or be a result of arthritis.

If you have any kind of joint surgery, physical therapy likely will be necessary to increase the strength of muscles that support the joint that was operated on and to help the joint – and you – function optimally afterwards.

Although you probably will want to consult your doctor about physical therapy, in most cases, you won't need a referral to consult a PT. If your problem is relatively minor, a session or two with a PT may provide the information you need to begin an effective exercise program. On the other hand, if your arthritis is severe and affects several joints, or if you are having major surgery such as total hip replacement, you may need regular, frequent sessions – at least for a while.

OCCUPATIONAL THERAPY

Similar to physical therapy, the goal of occupational therapy is to help you function better with arthritis. Instead of exercise, occupational therapy focuses on different ways of doing things or using devices to help you manage specific household, self-care and job-related activities. An occupational therapist (OT) is trained in joint-protection techniques and how to design or prescribe splints and assistive devices.

If arthritis makes it difficult for you to do such tasks as brush your teeth, shower, get dressed, drive a car, work on a computer, cook or fold laundry, an OT may help.

Similarly, if arthritis makes it difficult for you to pursue leisure activities, such as arts and crafts or photography, an OT may be able to recommend or devise new ways of holding a camera, carrying equipment, or cutting, gluing or painting craft projects.

An occupational therapist may recommend special devices – such as long-handled reachers, spring-loaded scissors, built-up brush handles or keys, or computer arm rests – to help you with your activities. The OT may prescribe or design splints or braces to protect joints and hold them in proper position while you are working or resting.

Braces and splints

Braces and splints are devices used to support or stabilize a joint. Braces and splints are made from an array of materials, such as metal, plastic, cloth and moldable foam. They may be used after surgery, for example, to hold a joint in position while it fuses following arthrodesis, or to support a replaced knee until the supporting muscles have been sufficiently strengthened to do the job through physical therapy. In some cases, they are prescribed to stabilize a joint that is causing disability.

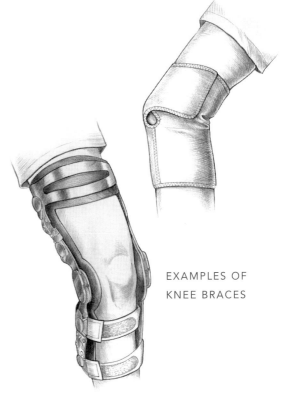

EXAMPLES OF KNEE BRACES

Splints and braces may be worn to position a joint in a way that helps prevent further irritation or injury to a joint or the soft tissues surrounding it. Wrist splints commonly are used for this purpose. Wrist splints may be especially helpful for people with rheumatoid arthritis in the wrist or with carpal tunnel syndrome, a condition in which the soft tissues in the wrist swell and compress the nerve running the length of the arm to the palm, causing numbness or tingling in the fingers.

Some people find it helpful to wear braces or splints during the day as they go about their activities; others prefer to wear them at night to keep their joints from bending awkwardly while they sleep. Some people wear them 24 hours a day.

In most cases, your physician or therapist prescribing the splint or brace will give you instructions on when to use it. Most health professionals advise not wearing a splint or brace around the clock unless specifically told to do so, because constantly holding a joint in one position long-term could potentially lead to permanently diminished range of motion.

Another type of splint, made for the fingers, can help prevent hand deformity. Such splints may be made of silver-colored metal and look more like jewelry than medical devices. Ask your doctor or physical therapist for information about finger splints.

Braces and splints can be store-bought or custom designed and made by a physical or occupational therapist or an orthotist, a person who specializes in making braces, splints and similar devices.

The Arthritis Foundation distributes a free brochure called "Bracing and Osteoarthritis" that has a great deal of information about braces and splints. Call 800-283-7800 to request this brochure and other information about arthritis.

JOINT PROTECTION

In the course of each day, sore, damaged joints are taxed by all of the activities you must perform just to maintain a home, prepare a meal, perform a job, practice good hygiene or complete your daily tasks. We stress our joints each time we walk, lift, grip, hold, twist, cut, write, reach, brush, bend or stir. By knowing how to protect our joints, however, we can use them in ways that avoid excess stress. Here are a few things you might try:

- **Pay attention to joint position.** This means using joints in the best way to avoid excess stress on them, such as using larger or stronger joints to carry things. For instance, you might carry bags by using your forearms or palms instead of your fingers.
- **Use assistive devices.** Devices, such as canes, crutches and walkers, can reduce stress on your hips and knees. Ballpoint pens with built-up handles can protect finger joints and make it easier to write. Long handles and reachers may spare shoulders when you need an item from a high shelf. Lightweight items, such as paper cups or plastic dishes, are easier to carry, and lightweight items, such as small, light vacuum cleaners, are easier to maneuver, making it easier to keep house.
- **Control your weight.** Excess pounds add

Helpful Hints for Using Hot and Cold

Using heat and cold treatments can be an easy and effective way to reduce pain, inflammation and stiffness. There is a right way and a wrong way to do it. Follow the suggestions below to get the greatest benefits from your hot and cold treatment and to reduce the risk of harm to the skin and underlying tissue.

- Use heat or cold for only 15 to 20 minutes at a time.

- Avoid using treatments that are extremely hot or cold.

- Always put a towel between your skin and the hot or cold pack.

- Don't use creams, rubs or lotions on your skin with a cold or hot treatment.

- To prevent burns, turn off your heating pad before going to sleep.

- Use an electric blanket or mattress pad. Turn it up before you get out of bed to help ease morning stiffness. Follow the directions on the blanket or pad carefully to ensure safety.

- Use a hot-water bottle to keep your feet, back or hands warm.

- Consult your doctor or physical therapist before using cold packs if you have poor circulation, vasculitis or Raynaud's phenomenon.

- As with any treatment, follow the advice of your health-care professional when using these methods.

excess stress to joints of the knees, hips and feet. If you have knee OA, losing weight may spare your joint some stress and reduce pain.

For more suggestions on ways to protect your joints, read *The Arthritis Foundation's Tips for Good Living with Arthritis*, a new book full of joint-protection tips and ideas for using assistive devices. Order this book by calling 800/207-8633 or log on to www.arthritis.org and browse the Arthritis Foundation's Arthritis Store for this and other books about arthritis.

HOT AND COLD TREATMENTS

Heat and cold treatments are easy methods you can use at home to reduce the pain and stiffness of arthritis. Cold packs can numb the painful area and reduce inflammation and swelling. They are especially good for joint pain caused by a flare of arthritis. Heat, on the other hand, relaxes muscles and stimulates blood circulation.

Heat and cold can be applied to joints in a number of ways. Cold may be applied with commercially available cold packs that can be

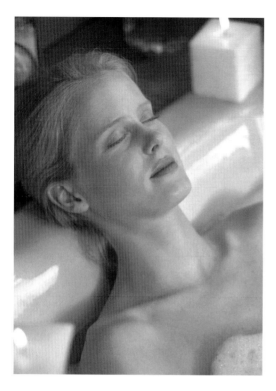

placed in your freezer and refrozen, as needed. You can make your own cold pack by wrapping a towel around a bag of frozen peas or a sealable sandwich bag filled with ice.

Heat treatments may be dry or moist. Dry heat sources include heat lamps or heating pads. Moist heat sources include warm baths, washcloths soaked in warm water and paraffin baths, which involve placing the affected joint, usually those of the hand or wrist, into a container of melted paraffin, which adheres to skin, and provides warmth.

Before using either hot or cold, be sure your skin is dry and free from cuts and sores. If you have visible skin damage, don't use cold or heat, especially paraffin baths. After using heat or cold,

carefully dry the skin and check for purplish-red skin or hives, which may indicate the treatment was too strong. Allow your skin to return to normal temperature and color before using heat or cold again.

For some helpful tips on using heat and cold safely, see "Helpful Hints for Using Hot and Cold" on page 135.

WATER THERAPY

You know how good it can feel to soak in a warm tub, especially when your joints are aching, your muscles are cramping and you're feeling downright miserable. It turns out that being in water not only feels good, it's good for you. Studies have shown that the benefits of applying heat can include muscle relaxation and decreased pain and stiffness. Immersing your body in warm water is an especially good way to apply heat to many parts of the body all at once.

By allowing your muscles to relax, warm water also provides an excellent environment for exercise. Water also may act as resistance to help build muscle strength during exercise, and the buoyancy of water supports the joints, making exercise easier and allowing you to move in ways that you can't when out of the water.

If you find that pain and stiffness are worst in the morning, soaking and performing gentle exercises in a tub, whirlpool bath or warm shower upon arising can help you get ready to take on your daily activities. If pain increases throughout the day, a warm soak before bedtime might make it easier to get to sleep. Be aware that some people find soaking before bed-

How To Do Self-Massage

You bump your elbow or close a cabinet door on your finger. What is your first response? If you're like most people, you probably rub the painful area. And when you do, it probably feels a little better, at least for a while.

With a little instruction and practice, a similar type of rubbing – called self-massage – can help relieve the pain of arthritis. Your hands can benefit, too, because they'll get a workout during the process.

If you'd like try self-message, here are a few suggestions for getting started:

- **Get professional advice.** A massage therapist can show you some techniques to use.

- **Warm up before you start.** A warm bath or shower can relax you, make your hands more limber and improve circulation.

- **Create a healing environment.** Find a warm, quiet place without distractions. For some people, music can help create a relaxing environment.

- **Use a little lotion.** Using a little oil or lotion can help your hands glide over your body. A lightly scented massage oil can be soothing to your body – and your spirit.

- **Consider an appliance.** If your hands are affected to the point where self-massage is painful or impossible, or if limited range of motion makes it difficult to reach painful joints, try a vibrating massage appliance. Be sure to follow package instructions and limit the use to a few minutes at a time.

- **Be firm, but gentle.** Use firm, gentle strokes and pressure, especially over the joints where skin and muscle layers are thin. Pressing too hard can irritate your skin and the joint or muscle you are trying to help.

time to be stimulating, and this practice keeps them awake. If that's the case with you, limit your use of warm water to the afternoon and early evening hours.

MASSAGE THERAPY

Aside from medication, surgery and physical therapy, massage may be one of the most widely used arthritis treatments. Although it is not well-studied for arthritis, many people report significant benefits in terms of pain and relaxation. Many doctors recommend it for their patients and some even have massage therapists working in their clinics. Although there are many forms of massage, the type most people are familiar with is Swedish massage, a full-body treatment

THE GOUT EXCEPTION

Although most forms of arthritis probably are influenced very little by the types of foods you eat, there is one notable exception: gout. Gout occurs when a bodily waste product called uric acid builds up in the blood and deposits as crystals in the joints, causing joints to become hot, swollen and excruciatingly painful.

While medication is needed to treat gout in many people, proper diet and weight loss can help keep the disease under control. If you have gout, your doctor probably will advise you to limit alcohol consumption to no more than one or two drinks a day and to avoid such foods as organ meats, sardines, anchovies and fish roe.

It's also important that you stay well-hydrated, by drinking eight 8-ounce glasses of nonalcoholic, decaffeinated liquids per day.

that involves stroking or kneading the top layers of muscles with oils or lotions.

Other forms of massage include:

- Deep tissue massage, in which the massage therapist uses fingers, thumbs and elbows to put strong pressure on deep muscle or tissue layers to relieve chronic tension.
- Neuromuscular massage (also called trigger point therapy), in which the therapist applies pressure with the fingers to certain spots that can trigger pain in other parts of the body.
- Myofascial release, a type of massage that involves applying slow, steady pressure to relieve tension in the fascia, or thin tissue around the muscles.

Although massage therapy generally is safe, as with any therapy, there are some precautions. For example, you should never have massage on an inflamed joint or on skin that is broken or infected. Let your massage therapist know if you have other health problems, including circulatory problems.

If you think you might be interested in massage, consult your physician, physical therapist or other health professional who may be able to refer you to a massage therapist with experience in your particular condition.

DIET AND WEIGHT LOSS

Although anecdotal reports of food-allergy-induced arthritis abound, research has shown that food sensitivities rarely play a role in arthritis. That's not to say that what you eat doesn't matter. For optimal health — whether you have arthritis or not — it's important to consume a healthful diet that is rich in vitamins and minerals and low in saturated fats and calories.

Most rheumatologists advise their patients to follow a diet such as those recommended by the American Heart Association (online at www. americanheart.org) or American Cancer Society (online at www.cancer.org), both of which emphasize fruits, vegetables and grains. Consuming plenty of calcium-rich products, including fortified juices and low-fat dairy products, keeps bones strong, reducing your risk of osteoporosis.

In addition, people with inflammatory forms of arthritis, such as rheumatoid arthritis or ankylosing spondylitis, may benefit from changing the types of fats and oils in their diets. Safflower, sunflower and corn oil, as well as fats in meat and poultry, may contribute to inflammation; olive, canola, flaxseed oils and cold water fish oils may help reduce inflammation.

Some people believe that certain foods make their arthritis worse. If you suspect a food is aggravating your arthritis, it can't hurt to eliminate that food from your diet for a few weeks and observe what happens. But doctors advise against cutting out entire groups of foods (such as all dairy products, all green vegetables or all fruits, for example), which could leave you with nutritional deficiencies. It's also important that you not stop taking your medications, even if you believe you have eliminated a problematic food. Because arthritis can come and go, it's difficult to be certain if a food really is having an effect on your disease. Neglecting your medical treatment while pursuing problem foods can leave you vulnerable to a flare of arthritis or irreparable joint damage.

Whether diet has a direct effect on arthritis or not, a healthy diet can help you manage your weight and take off and keep off excess pounds that are hard on your weight-bearing joints. A proper diet can reduce your risk of cardiovascular disease and cancer, either of which could be devastating, especially if you have arthritis.

The Food Guide Pyramid

As we learned, losing pounds if necessary, or maintaining your weight if it is appropriate, requires a balanced lifestyle of regular exercise and proper diet. Consult your doctor or a registered dietitian if you need advice on losing weight. A good general guideline for a balanced daily food intake is the USDA's Food Guide Pyramid, a visual diagram of the government agency's recommended healthy diet. The foods at the base of the pyramid should make up the bulk of your diet, the foods in the middle should be eaten in moderate quantities, and the foods at the very top of the pyramid should be eaten sparingly. The suggested diet emphasizes building your daily food intake on a base of low-fat,

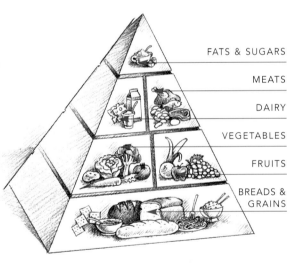

FOLLOWING THE FOOD GUIDE PYRAMID CAN HELP YOU EAT A WELL-BALANCED DIET THAT CONSISTS PRIMARILY OF GRAINS, FRUITS AND VEGETABLES.

high-fiber breads, grains and complex carbo-hydrates; eating several servings a day of fruits and vegetables; including moderate amounts of lean proteins such as fish, meats and poultry; eating moderate servings of dairy products, which add calcium; and eating small amounts of fats, sugars and oils.

Many packaged food products, such as cereals and crackers, now carry the colorful pyramid on their boxes. See page 139 for an example of this helpful pyramid to follow in your daily eating routine.

TRANSCUTANEOUS ELECTRICAL NERVE STIMULATION (TENS)

If your pain is severe and doesn't respond to medication or other non-medication therapies, and if it is localized to the spine or a single hip or knee, you may be a candidate for transcutaneous electrical nerve stimulation (TENS). As its name suggests, TENS is a technique that uses electrical stimulation to the nerves to block pain signals to the brain.

In administering TENS, your doctor will place electrodes on your skin near the painful area. The electrodes will be attached to a small, battery-operated box that emits low-level electrical energy. When the box emits its energy, you will receive a low-level shock that gives a tingling sensation and, if all goes well, some temporary relief from your pain.

TENS doesn't work for everyone, and it is expensive and not appropriate for widespread pain. For some people, however, it provides at least temporary relief when it may seem that nothing else helps.

STRESS REDUCTION

In addition to the disease process, one of the biggest factors in arthritis pain is stress. Being in pain is stressful and being under stress can add to your pain. Because stress and pain go hand-in-hand, there is not a clear line between stress-reduction therapies and pain-reduction therapies. Anything you do to ease pain will help ease the stress, and anything you do to ease stress has the potential to ease your pain.

Although this chapter primarily discusses methods used for pain relief, some of these methods may work equally well for stress. For example, you may get – or give yourself – a massage as a way to ease pain and relax. Similarly, you may take a walk or a yoga class or soak in a warm tub to relieve stress and pain.

In Chapter 11, we'll discuss some of activities and techniques you may pursue purely for relaxation. These activities may have the pleasant side effect of easing your pain.

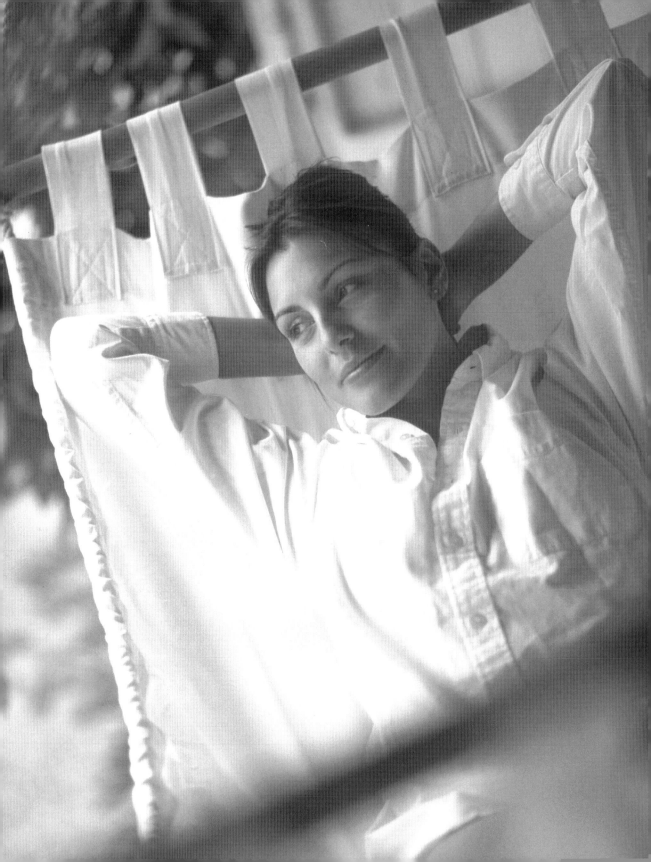

Reducing Stress

11

CHAPTER 11: REDUCING STRESS

Nobody lives completely free from stress. In our fast-paced, have-it-all, do-it-all society, stress is a daily problem in many people's lives. When you feel stressed, your muscles become tense. Muscle tension can, in turn, increase your pain and limit your physical abilities, which can lead to depression. A vicious cycle of stress, pain, limited/lost abilities and depression may develop.

If you have arthritis, you're not immune to the same kind of stressors that affect everyone else. In addition, you probably will have some stresses that healthy people don't, such as having to make important treatment decisions, needing to rely on other people more than in the past, making changes in your lifestyle and favorite activities because of limited abilities, or seeing your appearance changed by the effects of the disease. None of these stressors are easy to deal with, but learning how to manage your stress can make it a little easier and help break the stress–pain–limited/lost abilities–depression cycle.

If stress is affecting your life and your health, learning to relax may be one of the most helpful things you can do for yourself, but you must understand that relaxing involves more than just kicking back and watching TV for an hour or two before bedtime. It involves becoming aware of what causes you stress and what you can do to eliminate the stressor or change your reaction to it.

For example, if you have young children and having a messy house causes you to be stressed, teaching your children to clean up after them-selves, limiting their number of toys and enlisting your spouse to clean up may help eliminate the stressor (a messy house). Changing your reaction to the stressor would be admitting to yourself that children make messes and insisting on a spotless house is not only unrealistic, but may also needlessly affect your health.

The first step in easing stress in your life is to recognize what causes you stress and how you respond to it. Although that sounds obvious, the causes of stress aren't always clear-cut. For example, you may attribute a stress-related stomachache to something you ate. Or you may think that a stress headache was caused by a medication, sinus congestion or any number of factors – until you notice that you get one every time you face a stressful situation. To help yourself identify your stressors and your responses to them, try keeping a diary using the model on page 145.

STRESS REDUCTION AND RELAXATION TECHNIQUES

As troublesome as stress is, something as simple as taking time to daydream or write in a journal can help reduce your stress – and may even have beneficial effects on your pain and your disease.

Keeping a Stress Diary

An important first step to eliminating stress is to identify what causes it and how you respond, physically and emotionally. By keeping a daily stress diary, you should start to discover a pattern of stressors and symptoms. You will see how

A Sample Stress Diary

Date	Time	Cause of Stress	Physical Symptoms	Emotional Symptoms
4/18	7 a.m.	Getting kids off to school	Fast heartbeat, tightness of neck	feel rushed, disorganized
4/18	8 a.m.	Stuck in traffic	headache, heart beating faster, legs aching	frustrated, angry at being late
4/18	9 a.m.	Meeting presentation	fast heartbeat, dry throat, clammy palms	anxious, nervous
4/18	6:35 p.m.	Cooking Dinner	Headache, jaw tightening	Feel overwhelmed
4/18	8 p.m.	Watching TV w/Kids	Fast heartbeat	Angry; kids argued to watch cop shows

a stressor causes both physical and emotional reactions. Then you can begin to address your stress by using some of the techniques in this book. See "A Sample Stress Diary" on this page for an example you can follow.

Relaxation Techniques

Relaxation techniques help you deal more calmly and effectively with life's stresses. Following are a few common techniques that might help:

Deep breathing. To practice deep breathing, sit in a comfortable chair with your feet on the floor and your arms at your sides. Close your eyes and breathe in deeply, saying to yourself, "I am….," then slowly breathe out, while saying, "…relaxed."

Continue to breathe slowly, silently repeating something to yourself such as, "My hands …are warm; my feet …are warm; my breathing …is deep and smooth; my heartbeat …is calm and steady; I feel calm …and at peace."

Always coordinate the words you say with your breathing.

Distraction. Distraction involves training your mind to focus on something other than your stress. This does not mean that you will ignore your stress, only that you choose not to dwell on it. When you anticipate a stressful situation, such as driving in heavy traffic or having a joint injection, prepare yourself for the stress and how you will handle it. Make plans for what you will do once the stressful situation has passed, because although it may seem at the time as if the problem will last forever, it will pass. By thinking of something else, you can take your mind off what is causing you stress.

Guided imagery. Like distraction, guided imagery helps take your focus off your stress. To practice guided imagery, close your eyes, take a deep breath and hold it for several seconds. Breathe out slowly, feeling your body relax as you do. Think about a place you have been where you felt safe and comfortable. Imagine it in as much detail as possible. Imagine the sounds you heard – of waves against the sand, seagulls calling overhead, children laughing on the beach. Imagine the way it felt, smelled and tasted – the saltwater on your lips, the soft sand beneath your feet, the ocean breeze blowing through your hair. Recapture the positive feelings you had when you were there and keep them in your mind. Take several deep breaths and enjoy feeling calm and peaceful before you open your eyes.

Progressive relaxation. Progressive relaxation is a therapy in which the body's muscles, from head to toe, are progressively tensed and then relaxed. Progressive relaxation is a popular form of stress management.

To practice progressive relaxation, first close your eyes and take a deep breath, filling your chest and breathing all the way down to your abdomen. Breathe out, letting your stress flow out with the air. Beginning with your feet and calves, slowly tense your muscles. Hold for several seconds, then release and relax the muscles. Slowly work your way through your major muscle groups using the same technique, until you have tensed and relaxed the muscles of your neck and face. Continue breathing deeply and enjoy the feeling of relaxation before opening your eyes.

Visualization. One of the most stressful aspects of a chronic disease such as arthritis is that it can make you feel as if your life is out of your control. Visualization helps reduce that stress by allowing you to imagine yourself anyway you like, doing anything you want to do. In other words, you are in control of the scenario. Also, by focusing on doing the things you like, you are not focusing on the things that cause you stress.

One form of visualization involves concentrating on pleasant scenes from your past or creating new situations in your mind. For example, you might try to remember every detail of a special vacation or of your first date with your spouse. Alternatively, you could imagine yourself taking your dream vacation or having a date with an attractive movie star.

Another form of visualization involves thinking of symbols that represent the pain or stress in different parts of your body. For example you might imagine that a painful knee or tense shoulder muscles are bright red, then imagine yourself making the red fade or change to cool, soothing blue. You might imagine your pain as a little monster that you could put in a trash can and shut the lid or wrap in a small box that you drop into a mailbox – with no return address, of course. For some specific mental exercises to help you relax, try the following techniques.

Sample Relaxation Exercises

For the following exercises, you'll never have to break a sweat or even leave your easy chair, because your mind is doing the work. The most important part of these exercises is that you be comfortable. Pick a place, get quiet and comfortable and start to focus on your breathing. Imagine that fresh air is coming in and tension is being released with every breath. Then try one or more of the exercises described below. Pick a favorite exercise to save for times when you're feeling stressed.

"Pain drain." Feel within your body and note where you experience pain or tension. Imagine that the pain or tension is turning into a liquid substance. This heavy liquid flows down through your body and through your fingers and toes. Allow the pain to drain from your body in a steady flow. Now, imagine that a gentle stream flows down over your head . . . and further dissolves the pain . . . into a liquid that continues to drain away. Enjoy the sense of comfort and well-being that follows.

"Disappearing pain." Notice any tension or pain that you are experiencing. Imagine that the pain takes the form of an object, or of several objects. It can be fruit, pebbles, crystals or anything else that comes to mind. Pick up each piece of pain, one at a time, and place it in a magic box.

As you drop each piece into the box, it dissolves into nothingness. Now, again survey your body to see if any pieces remain, and remove them. Imagine that your body is lighter now, and allow yourself to experience a feeling of comfort and well-being. Enjoy this feeling of tranquility and repose.

"Healing potion." Imagine you are in a drugstore that is stocked with bottles and jars of exotic potions. Each potion has a special magical quality. Some are of pure white light, others are lotions, balms and creams, and yet others contain healing vibrations. As you survey the many potions, choose one that appeals to you. It may even have your name on the container. Open the container and cover your body with that magical potion. As you apply it, let any pain or tension slowly melt away, leaving you with a feeling of comfort and well-being. Imagine that you place the container in a special spot and that it continually renews its contents for future use.

Biofeedback

Imagine being able to lower your heart rate or blood pressure or raise the temperature of your cold, achy hands at will. Using a process called biofeedback, the idea is not as far-fetched as it sounds. In fact, biofeedback can help you control many body processes that previously were considered to be out of conscious control. Biofeedback also can help you control your body's response to stress.

What is biofeedback? In a nutshell, it's the use of electronic instruments to measure body function and feed this back to you so that you can learn to control them. With practice, you can learn to control almost any body process that can be measured.

In a biofeedback session, sensors are attached to the part of the body being monitored – such as your cold hands or a stiff muscle in your neck – and then connected to an electronic instrument, such as computer. The instruments might read your skin temperature, electrical signals produced by your muscles, your heart rate, or your brain waves.

The practitioner conducting biofeedback will teach you some relaxation techniques, such as visualization, to influence your subconscious body processes. As you practice these mental techniques, the instruments show with sound, light or other signals the effects that your thoughts are having on your body. Eventually, you will learn what mental relaxation techniques to use to get the physical effect you want, and you will be able to do them on your own without the equipment.

Keeping a Journal

When you were an adolescent, you may have found that confiding in a diary or journal – about a fight with your best friend, exam-time anxiety or a breakup with your latest sweetheart, for example – helped defuse some of the emotions that came with a stressful or hurtful experience. Research shows that a variation on the writing you may have done then can help you cope with the stress that comes with arthritis now. Furthermore, one recent study of people with RA showed that those who regularly wrote about their most stressful life events experienced a 28 percent reduction in overall disease activity.

Although it was just a single study, it substantiates long-held speculation that stress can contribute to disease activity. It also shows that reducing stress – specifically by writing about emotionally painful events – may decrease arthritis severity.

At the very least, keeping a journal can help you identify situations that cause you stress, and identifying stressors is the first step to finding ways to cope with or eliminate them. On page 145, you'll find a sample stress diary that you can use as a model to get you started. If you prefer a more free-form approach, try some of the following suggestions to begin your journaling:

- **Choose your pen and paper.** Find a spiral notebook or blank book with lots of open space to begin writing. Or, find a decorative notebook or journal at your local bookstore or art supply store. Select a pen or pencil with a comfortable grip that is easy to hold. If you prefer, write your journal on your computer.

- **Don't worry about penmanship or spelling.** A journal should be for your eyes only, so you won't need to impress anyone with neat writing, proper grammar and expert spelling. Stopping to look up a word in the dictionary or contemplate grammatical issues can interfere with self-expression.

- **Choose the time and place.** Don't try to write in your journal while you watch TV or stir a pot of soup on the stove. Pick a place without distractions and a time when you won't be interrupted. Focus entirely on your writing.

- **Don't hold back.** Don't be afraid to express your emotions – all of them. Your journal won't judge you and no one else will have to see it.

- **Pick your style.** You may wish to write about

events as if you were a newspaper reporter covering your life, or you may wish to write your feelings in a letter – aren't there a few things you would like to tell arthritis? You may find one style that you'll want to stick with, or you may vary your style from day to day. It's your book – do what works for you.

- **Get help if you need it.** Writing can stir painful feelings, which themselves may be difficult to deal with – that's part of the process of letting go of pain and stress. If you feel you need help coping with the feelings that writing ar-

ouses, consult a counselor or minister. Sometimes taking your journal along with you to counseling – and reading selected passages aloud – can help your counselor help you.

The Arthritis Foundation publishes a journal specifically designed for people with arthritis. *Toward Healthy Living: A Wellness Journal* is a spiral-bound, glossy journal with inspiring quotes in the borders of pages, as well as charts to track daily changes in pain and mood. To order, call 800/207-8633 or log on to www.arthritis.org.

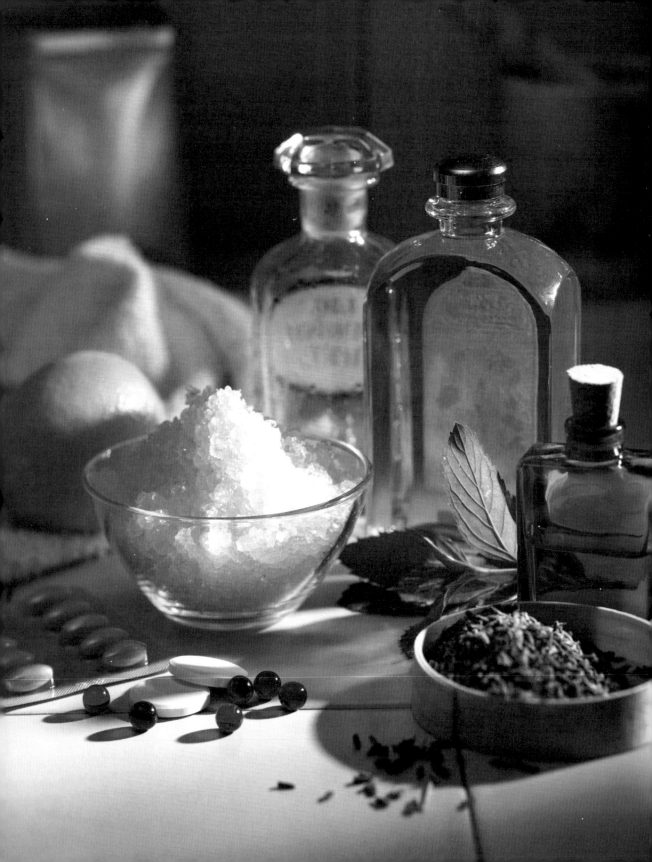

Alternative Therapies
for Arthritis

12

CHAPTER 12:
ALTERNATIVE THERAPIES FOR ARTHRITIS

While most of the treatments and therapies discussed in this book have been scientifically studied and prescribed or are used routinely by the medical profession, many of the therapies people with arthritis try and even swear by are not backed by scientific research. These therapies commonly are referred to as alternative or complementary therapies and include such treatments as herbs and nutritional supplements, magnets and copper bracelets.

Alternative and complementary therapies (also referred to as unproven remedies) are nothing new. In fact, many have their roots in ancient times. As people strive to take control of their own health care and to find natural alternatives to doctor-prescribed medications, the use of complementary and alternative therapies is increasing.

This growth may be especially noteworthy among people with painful, chronic diseases like arthritis for which there are no cures. If the medication your doctor prescribes isn't helping, you'd be tempted to try just about anything. And if you do try an alternative therapy, the tendency of arthritis symptoms to come and go or wax and wane may make it seem like the therapy is working. Whether or not this is true may be hard to determine.

Let's say, for example, you put on a copper bracelet and the swelling goes down in your wrist. Was the copper bracelet responsible or would the swelling have gone down anyway?

Or suppose you try a new nutritional supplement and discover that your joints are less painful and stiff. Did the nutritional supplement help or did your joints coincidentally get better?

Sometimes just the belief that a treatment will help is all it takes to bring some relief. Medical professionals refer to this as the *placebo effect* – a measurable effect on a person who has been given an inert substance or a fake therapy – and they suspect that it plays a big role in the effectiveness of many alternative therapies. The placebo effect may play a role in the seeming effectiveness of some alternative therapies in the relief of subjective symptoms like pain, fatigue or stiffness. In scientific studies of medications, the placebo effect is accounted for by not allowing patients (or the physician administering the study) to know whether they are getting the medication studied.

Fortunately, as alternative and complementary therapies gain acceptance among patients and physicians, they also are being put to the test scientifically. In the late 1990s, the federal government formed the National Center for Complementary and Alternative Medicine (NCCAM) at the National Institutes of Health to conduct and support clinical and basic research into complementary and alternative therapies. As doctors learn more about these therapies, the treatments may gain even wider acceptance.

In the meantime, if you want to try an unproven remedy, it's best to work closely with your physician and to learn as much about the therapy as you can before you try it. At the same time, understand that there is not a lot of good scientific information about many alternative therapies, so you'll be proceeding at your own risk. Although many alternative therapies claim to be natural, even natural remedies aren't always safe. Many natural things – arsenic, uranium and poison ivy, to name a few – have obvious toxicities. Because they haven't been well-studied, it is difficult to anticipate what side effects alternative therapies may have.

Be aware that such products as nutritional supplements may interact with your prescribed medications, either interfering with or adding to their action. Perhaps most dangerous, however, is the possibility that while using alternative remedies you may neglect the medical treatments your doctor prescribes – the ones that have proven benefits for people with arthritis.

In this chapter, we'll provide a brief overview of some of the most widely used or highly touted complementary and alternative therapies for arthritis. A more complete listing could easily fill a book. In fact, it has – *The Arthritis Foundation's Guide to Alternative Therapies*. The information in this chapter is expanded upon in that book, which features more in-depth information on these and many other alternative and complementary therapies. *The Arthritis Foundation's Guide to Alternative Therapies* is available by calling 800/207-8633, by visiting www.arthritis.org, or in all major bookstores.

NUTRITIONAL SUPPLEMENTS

The most commonly used alternative therapies are nutritional supplements. These are vitamins, herbs, minerals and animal compounds purported to promote good health. Once sold only in nutrition or health-food stores, these prod-

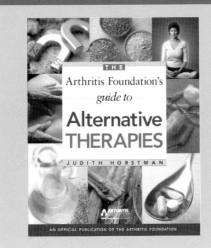

ucts now line the shelves of almost every pharmacy, supermarket and discount department store. Many are promoted and sold over the Internet and through multi-level marketing schemes. You may even find a shelf of them for sale in your doctor's office.

High accessibility, ease of use and promises of being all-natural often make nutritional supplements popular among people seeking relief from arthritis pain and other symptoms. Do they work? And are they safe? Here's what we know about some of the supplements that commonly are used for arthritis and related conditions:

Glucosamine

Glucosamine is one of the hottest nutritional supplements for osteoarthritis – and maybe with good reason. Although it is not the cure for arthritis as some have claimed, it does appear to ease the pain and stiffness of osteoarthritis. In fact, there's a growing body of evidence that this supplement – which is extracted from crab, shrimp and lobster shells – may ease pain just as well as NSAIDs. There's even speculation that it may help repair damaged cartilage, but that claim has not been proved.

The National Institutes of Health currently is sponsoring a large study of glucosamine that, over the next few years, should yield a better understanding of the supplement's role in treating OA. Since the supplement is safe for most people, if you can afford it, you may find it worthwhile to give it a try.

If you have diabetes, however, you may want to consult your doctor before taking glucosamine because it could potentially raise blood sugars.

Chondroitin Sulfate

In the body, naturally existing chondroitin sulfate is thought to draw fluid into the cartilage to help give it its elasticity and slow cartilage breakdown. The supplement, which is derived from cattle trachea, often is taken with glucosamine to ease the symptoms of osteoarthritis. Like glucosamine, chondroitin appears to be without serious side effects, so you may want to give a try. But be prepared to wait for results. It can take two or more months for this supplement's effects to show.

Boswellia

Derived from a tree from Asia, boswellia (*boswellia serrata*) comes in a standardized extract of the gum oleoresin. In animal and test tube studies, boswellia inhibits leukotriene synthesis, which contributes to inflammation. But studies have failed to consistently show any relief from pain and inflammation in people with arthritis.

The most common side effects of boswellia are diarrhea, nausea or a rash. Otherwise, it is considered safe.

Cat's Claw

A vine that grows wild in the Peruvian Amazon, cat's claw (*uncaria tomentosa*) gets its name from its claw-shaped thorns. The vine has a long tradition as a treatment for inflammation and "bone pain." At least one animal study shows that cat's claw just might prevent inflammation and other cell damage. However, there have been no human studies to document its effectiveness or its safety.

Cetyl Myristoleate (CMO)

Although you may see this advertised as a quick cure for many forms of arthritis, there is no accepted scientific evidence so far that CMO helps any form of arthritis – at least in people.

CMO's fantastic claims stemmed from a 1993 study showing that injecting CMO into rats prevented them from developing arthritis. But one study on rats isn't reason enough to try a supplement that could be dangerous in people. Perhaps the most dangerous aspect of CMO is that some CMO vendors advise people considering the supplement to stop taking methotrexate and glucocorticoids first (explaining that these drugs could interfere with CMO's action). By giving up your regular medications you could be sustaining irreparable joint damage as you wait to see if CMO might work.

DHEA

Short for dehydroepiandrosterone, DHEA is a mild male hormone produced naturally by the body. DHEA supplements have been touted as a cure for everything from cancer to old age. Most of its claims haven't been proved; however, the hormone is showing promise as a therapy for lupus and is under FDA review for approval as a prescription drug. Although it's not exactly clear how DHEA works for lupus, it is believed to restore an imbalance of male and female hormones in women with lupus.

Because DHEA carries the risk of side effects, ranging from acne to reduced levels of HDL (good cholesterol), you should only use it under the supervision of a physician.

Dimethyl Sulfoxide (DMSO)

In the early 1960s, DMSO, a by-product of wood processing, was being hailed as a new therapy for all forms of arthritis. But studies of the substance were halted in the mid-'60s because high doses damaged the lens of the eye in animal studies. (No eye problems have been documented in human studies of DMSO.)

Today, DMSO is widely used in Russia and other countries for rheumatoid arthritis and osteoarthritis, but in the United States it has only one approved use – for a bladder condition called interstitial cystitis.

There is research that suggests DMSO can relieve pain and increase function for people with arthritis and that it may ease finger ulcers in scleroderma and relieve blood vessel constrictions in Raynaud's phenomenon. But the research is mixed. More studies are required to confirm DMSO's safety and effectiveness.

Echinacea

A North American wildflower, echinacea (*echinacea purpurea, echinacea augustifolia*) is one of the top-selling herbal products in the United States and Europe. The supplement has been touted as an immune system booster and as a treatment for a variety of ills, including the common cold.

Although echinacea has been widely studied, experts believe that much of the research is flawed. Although it could be useful against infections, experts say it could be harmful for people with autoimmune diseases, whose immune systems already may be overactive.

Kava Kava

A nonalcoholic drink from the root of the kava plant, kava kava has been shown to work as a relaxant, relieving anxiety, promoting muscle relaxation and easing pain. While it may be worth it to give kava kava a try, doctors warn against mixing it with tranquilizers, antidepressant medications or alcohol, which could multiply the drink's effects.

Melatonin

A naturally occurring hormone that controls your sleep/wake cycle and helps regulate reproductive hormones, melatonin is made by the pineal gland deep in the brain, and our bodies make less of it as we age. In recent years, melatonin supplements have been touted as an immune system-booster and a sleep aid. Because fibromyalgia is associated with sleep difficulties, there has been speculation that melatonin might help, but research on its role in fibromyalgia has produced conflicting results. Experts advise against using it – particularly if you have an autoimmune disease, such as lupus, that could be made worse by boosting immune system activity.

MSM

Though touted on the Internet as one of the newest cures for arthritis, so far there is no scientific evidence to prove the effectiveness of MSM (short for methyl sulfonyl methane). MSM is a sulfur compound formed in the breakdown of DMSO. In animal studies, MSM has reduced arthritis symptoms. So far, there have been no published human studies of MSM.

SAM-e

S-adenosylmethionine, or SAM-e (pronounced "sammy") for short, is a naturally occurring compound that is believed to improve joint mobility, relieve pain and ease depression. Although a number of European studies have shown that SAM-e relieves pain as effectively as several NSAIDs, in U.S. studies, SAM-e appeared to work for only mild pain.

Some studies have shown that SAM-e works as well as tricyclic antidepressants for depression – and with fewer side effects. One downside to SAM-e is its high cost. Any benefits last only as long as you take it.

HANDS-ON APPROACHES
Osteopathic Medicine

Although osteopathic medicine often is listed as a complementary therapy, osteopathic physicians (doctors of osteopathic medicine, or DOs) complete a training, certification and licensing program that is almost identical as that of a medical doctor, or MD. Osteopathic physicians may perform surgery and write prescriptions, and some specialize in rheumatology.

The primary difference between DOs and MDs is philosophy. Osteopathic physicians believe problems with the musculoskeletal system can affect our health in many ways and that illness can, in turn, upset the balance of this

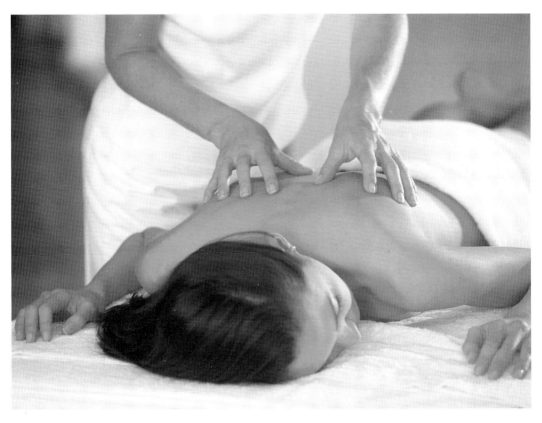

system. Improved blood flow, through osteopathic manipulation – of the muscles around the joints and spine and sometimes of the bones and tissues of the skull and spine – can help restore balance and relieve ills.

Osteopathic physicians may practice or recommend other alternative therapies, such as acupuncture or nutritional supplements.

Chiropractic

The third largest health-care profession in the country, chiropractic is used by more than 50 million Americans a year. Used primarily for back or neck pain following an injury or acci-

dent, chiropractic also is sought for other problems, including joint pain and stiffness related to arthritis. Chiropractic focuses on manual adjustments and manipulation of the spine.

Although the origins of spinal manipulation probably go back to antiquity, chiropractic as we know it began in the 1890s and is based on the theory that misalignment of the vertebrae in the spine (called subluxation) is the cause of almost all diseases, and that chiropractic adjustment of the spine is the cure.

Chiropractors complete a four-year program, focusing mainly on musculoskeletal issues, at one of 17 accredited chiropractic colleges. Some chiropractors do only spinal manipulation; others use a combination of treatments and techniques, including herbal and vitamin therapies, nutritional counseling and electrical stimulation.

Some studies have suggested that chiropractic may help relieve pain from OA of the knee or from fibromyalgia. If you have joints that are inflamed, deformed or weakened by arthritis, use caution when considering chiropractic, because manipulating the fragile joints could cause irreparable damage.

Massage

Rather than a single therapy, massage actually refers to more than 100 types of body work, each with a different technique and philosophy. Although they have different approaches, they offer similar physical and emotional benefits for people with arthritis and related conditions. For more information on massage, see page 137.

THE BENEFITS OF ALTERNATIVES

If you feel frustrated about what medical science has to offer, alternative and complementary therapies – when used wisely – may offer benefits over what you're getting from your doctor-prescribed medication. They also may give you the satisfaction that you are doing something for your disease. And some eventually may be scientifically proven to do what they claim. In fact, two supplements – glucosamine and chondroitin – are being studied in a major multicenter clinical trial. Another – DHEA – may soon be FDA-approved as a treatment for lupus.

Should you decide to proceed with an alternative or complementary therapy – and many people with arthritis do – it's important to understand as much as you can about the therapy. (For more on making the decision about alternatives, see "Evaluating Alternative and Complementary Therapies" on page 159.) It's also important not to abandon any proven therapies that you need to keep your disease in check – or to lose hope in scientific-based medicine.

Though medical science seems to move slowly when you're coping with a chronic painful disease, advances are occurring more rapidly than ever before. In Chapter 13, we'll discuss the potential they may hold for you – and even how you can play a role in getting new drugs on the market.

EVALUATING ALTERNATIVE THERAPIES

When you're considering a complementary or alternative therapy, it pays to be cautious. In your search for relief you may be willing to try something that helps nothing but the wallet of the person selling it. Never assume a product is safe just because it's natural.

Follow this advice if you think you might like to try an alternative or complementary therapy:

- **Know the facts.** Although drugs and other conventional therapies are monitored and regulated by government agencies like the FDA, such therapies as herbs, supplements and some other alternatives do not have to undergo that type of scrutiny to be marketed.
- **Use good judgment.** If a practitioner makes unrealistic claims, such as, "It will cure your arthritis," or suggests you discontinue your conventional treatments, consider it a strong warning that something is not right.
- **Seek out information.** Two good sources of information are *The Arthritis Foundation's Guide to Alternative Therapies*, available by calling 800/207-8633, by visiting www.arthritis.org, or at bookstores; and the National Center for Complementary and Alternative Medicine (NCCAM). For a free copy of the *Arthritis Today Supplement Guide*, call the Arthritis Foundation, 800/283-7800, or log on to the AF Web site.
- **Be a skeptic.** Beware of treatments that claim to work by a secret formula, say they are a cure or miraculous breakthrough, or are publicized in the backs of magazines, over the phone or through direct mail. Bona fide treatments are reported in medical journals.
- **Discuss it with your doctor.** Inform your doctor about any therapy you're trying, whether or not it is an alternative remedy. Your doctor can help you watch for and safeguard against side effects and possible negative interactions with medications you may be taking.
- **Consider the cost.** Some alternative therapies can be costly and most aren't covered by your health insurance. Read your policy closely to find what therapies are covered and under what circumstances. Then compare your ultimate cost of an alternative to that of a doctor-prescribed medication or treatment.
- **Proceed with caution.** If you decide to go through with an alternative treatment, seek out a qualified, licensed practitioner.
- **Don't abandon a treatment that works.** When starting an alternative therapy, don't stop taking the medication your doctor prescribes. Doing so could set you up for problems as diverse as heart problems or arthritis flares.

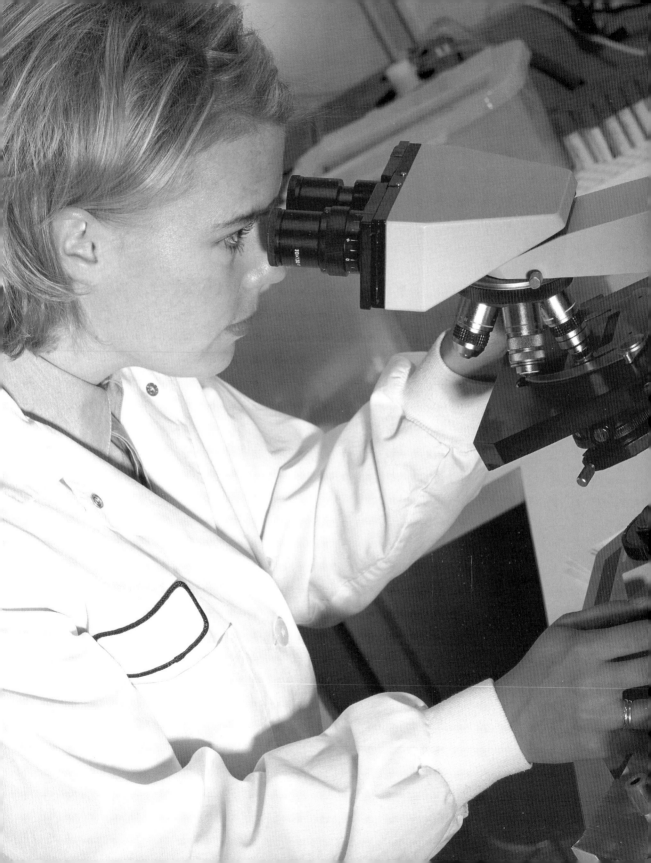

The Future of Arthritis

13

CHAPTER 13:
THE FUTURE OF ARTHRITIS

In this age of quick fixes, it's hard to understand why someone doesn't just come up with the cure for arthritis. After all, medical science can cure many other conditions. A bacterial infection that once might have proven fatal may now be eradicated with a course of antibiotics. An inflamed appendix that might have once ruptured and killed a person can now be removed surgically with no long-term detrimental effects.

Whether arthritis will someday join these medical success stories, no one can say. Certainly, finding a cure is a goal of research scientists, yet arthritis is many diseases – more than 100 complex diseases. It's not possible that one medication will cure all of the forms of the disease – or even ease all symptoms. And it's highly unlikely that a single medication could ever cure a single form of the disease or work for all people with a particular form of the disease.

Furthermore, even if scientists found a way to stop arthritis permanently, the "cure" would not undo any joint damage that has already taken place. That's why it's important to take advantage of all the good medications that are available today and to get proper treatment for your arthritis as soon as possible.

With today's medications, pain, joint deformity and organ damage are not inevitable consequences of arthritis-related diseases. Powerful immunosuppressive drugs such as cyclophosphamide can relieve inflammation and prevent damage to the kidneys that can occur in people with systemic lupus erythematosus, and high-blood pressure medications called angiotensin converting enzyme (ACE) inhibitors can prevent kidney damage that once meant death or a lifetime of dialysis for people with the arthritis-related disease systemic sclerosis, or systemic scleroderma.

For people with rheumatoid arthritis and perhaps other inflammatory forms of the disease, disease-modifying antirheumatic drugs can do just what their name suggests – modify the course of the disease and delay or inhibit joint damage. Furthermore, two biologic agents approved for rheumatoid arthritis, etanercept and infliximab, have been proven to delay or inhibit joint damage of rheumatoid arthritis.

UP-AND-COMING MEDICATIONS

In addition to all of the effective drugs that are available now, there are many others on the horizon that have caused great excitement. Some of them are still in early stages of clinical testing. Others may be approved in the near future.

Originally approved for cancer of the lymph nodes, rituximab is a monoclonal antibody that stops and destroys a type of white blood cell called B-lymphocytes. Because these lymphocytes are necessary to the production of rheumatoid factor and other self-directed antibodies in people with RA, British researchers reasoned that wiping out these B-lymphocytes might also rid the body of these damaging antibodies.

A very preliminary and small trial suggests those researchers just may be on to something. In 10 people treated with rituximab and then followed for six to 18 months, nine showed at least a 50 percent improvement in their disease symptoms. Larger studies of the drug, which are to begin in the near future, should tell us more about the drug's potential in treating RA.

One of the greatest areas of advancement in rheumatoid arthritis treatment will likely come in the area of biologic response modifiers. One biologic agent, referred to as a recombinant human interleukin-1 receptor antagonist (IL-1ra) or by its generic and trade names (anakinra, *Kineret*), works by blocking the inflammatory cytokine IL-1ra. At press time, the agent is currently under review by the FDA.

These are just a few of the many medications in the works that have the potential to improve the health and lives of people with one of the 100-plus forms of arthritis and related conditions. As this book goes to press, there are as many as 44 different drugs in clinical testing for arthritis and related conditions, according to the Pharmaceutical Research and Manufacturers of America. But getting those drugs to market takes time. And for every drug in clinical testing that makes it, there are four more that don't pass the test. (For more on the FDA approval process, see "How a Drug Makes It to Market on page" 168.)

STEM CELL TRANSPLANTATION

Despite the excitement of new medications, drugs are not the only new treatments on the horizon. One of the most exciting and promising treatments involves using existing immunosuppressive drugs in conjunction with autologous bone marrow or stem cell transplantation. Although the procedure is still highly experimental, it has been used with good results in some forms of arthritis.

The procedure involves removing so-called stem cells from a person's blood. Stem cells are 'mother cells' that have the capacity to expand and differentiate into many different types of cells, including infection-fighting T and B cells – the ones that go awry in some diseases.

After removing the stem cells, doctors administer high doses of immunosuppressive drugs to wipe out the patient's immune system. When existing immune cells are gone, the reserved stem cells are infused back into the patient, where, presumably, they will grow and differentiate into new immune system cells to replace the ones that were destroyed. So far, it appears that in some patients the new immune system created by a person's own stem cells does not malfunction the way the original immune system did.

In a recent study of seven women with lupus who had undergone stem cell transplants, all were relieved of signs of active lupus, and the functioning of their kidneys, hearts, lungs and immune systems – all of which had been affected by the disease – had returned to normal. Results in other diseases to date have not been as promising.

Despite such promising results in lupus, it's important to remember that the procedure is experimental, and it involves time, pain and risk. Between the time the original immune system

BEFORE YOU COMMIT TO A CLINICAL TRIAL

Before you sign up to participate in a study, it's essential to know what you're getting into. Here's how:

Speak to your doctor. Although your personal doctor may not be conducting the trial, he knows your medical condition more than any one else. Does he think this trial is a good idea? If so, why? If not, why not?

Read the fine print. Legally, the terms of participating in any study should be addressed in an informed consent form, which you'll be required to sign before you start. Don't hastily sign the form; ask to take it home and read over it carefully. You may even want to ask your spouse, a family member or a close friend to read it as well, in case you miss something.

Ask questions. If you still have questions after reading the informed consent form, don't hesitate to ask the doctor or other health-care professionals administering the study.

Here are some questions you might ask:

- What is the main purpose of the study?
- Are there any health risks involved?
- Do I have to stop taking my current medication(s)?
- What are the possible benefits?
- What happens if the study treatment harms me?
- Do I have the option of continuing the study treatment after the trial is over?
- Do I have to pay anything to take part?
- Will I be paid to take part?

Although you should do your best to follow the physician's instructions once you are in a trial (deviating from protocol could interfere with the accuracy of the study's results), you should never feel obligated to stay in a trial if you are uncomfortable about it. You have the right to leave the study at any time without it influencing your future medical care – regardless of what consent forms you have signed.

---

is destroyed and when the new stem cells start to create a new one (about a month) you would have to be hospitalized in a sterile room to avoid the risk of infection, because during that time – when you, in effect, have no immune system – any infection could prove fatal.

Nevertheless, if your disease is active and severely affects your life, any promising procedure may be worth investigating. As yet, stem cell transplantation is available only to people enrolled in clinical studies and reserved for the most severe cases of disease which have not be helped by any other measures.

Even these therapies are just the tip of the iceberg. As scientists learn more about the genetics of the different forms of arthritis, other factors that contribute to the diseases and individuals' responses to those factors, new treatments will emerge and doctors will be able to apply them early with increasingly better control. At any time there may be as many as a dozen or more new treatments in late stages of clinic testing for arthritis-related diseases. Each has the potential to be an improvement in some way over the drugs we have now, for at least some people.

YOU CAN PLAY A ROLE IN RESEARCH

What you might not know is that as a person with arthritis, you have an opportunity to play a role in the development of and testing of new treatments. Each year, thousands of people do, by enrolling in what are called clinical trials. A clinical trial is a carefully designed study of a potential new drug, medical treatment or medical device on a group of people with a particular condition. These studies, which are required for a treatment to be approved by the FDA for marketing, are typically funded by the manufacturer of the drug or device being tested. Without people like you, there could be no studies – and thus no new arthritis treatments.

Taking part in a clinical trial offers several potential benefits both to yourself and others in similar situations. First, taking part in a trial may allow you to receive cutting-edge medications and treatments before anyone else does, usually free of charge. Usually during the course of the study, any medical care associated with the study will be covered as well. You may even have access to a special place to sign in at the doctor's office and the assurance of being seen quickly by the

doctor. Some clinical trials may also pay a stipend to cover expenses such as mileage to the doctor's office, parking or meals en route.

Even if a study doesn't benefit you personally, your contribution to it will help add to knowledge of arthritis and perhaps help improve the lives of others with the disease.

As with any treatment – in fact, anything in life – there are also some potential drawbacks to participating in a trial. For one, you may not receive the new treatment being tested. In every clinical trial, a new treatment is compared to an existing treatment and/or a placebo (a "sham" procedure or pill without active ingredients).

That means you have chance – sometimes as high as 50/50 – of being in the other group. Also, because you may be receiving a new treatment that hasn't been used widely or for long, there is no way of knowing, with certainty, what the long-term effects of treatment might be. Furthermore, taking part in a trial for one drug may require that you stop taking a drug that has been helpful to you. For all of those reasons, most doctors should advise against taking part in a clinical trial if you are doing well with the medication you are taking.

Even if you choose not to take your chances with a new medical treatment, there are still ways you can contribute to research. One opportunity is by taking part in genetic registries. This is a process in which a researcher takes a blood sample and then compares your genes to those of people with and without the disease to look for similar and dissimilar genetic factors.

Another way to help arthritis research is by taking part in epidemiological studies, in which

Identifying Good Research

When it comes to reports about arthritis research, how can you separate the good from the bad or useless? A good starting point is to evaluate all you read by using the following criteria:

Consider the source:

Was it published in a peer-reviewed journal? The most reliable studies are those published in reputable journals and that have been reviewed by other doctors in the field prior to publication. Vague references to being scientifically tested may mean nothing.

Who did the research?

Was the person conducting the research from an institution you have heard of? Does the article say who funded the study? Research funded by the Arthritis Foundation or National Institutes of Health, for example, is usually reliable.

Who was studied?

While the research may good, it may mean nothing for you if the people in the study were in a different situation from yours. In other words, a new drug that looks promising in treating 100 women with rheumatoid arthritis may be of no use for a man who has osteoarthritis.

Have you seen similar reports elsewhere?

When evaluating a report in a magazine or newspaper or on a Web site, check around and see if you see similar information elsewhere. When writing about technical medical information, it's easy for a writer to get facts wrong. If you see consistent reports in several locations, however, it's more likely to be correct.

a researcher may ask you questions about diet, exercise and other lifestyle factors, for example, that may play a role in a certain form of arthritis. Some studies involve filling out periodic questionnaires.

If you think you might like to participate in a clinical trial, consult your physician. He might be aware of a trial for which you would be a candidate. In fact, he may be conducting such a trial himself.

Much of the clinical research that leads to the approval of new arthritis medications is conducted by rheumatologists, both in major medical centers and small, private practices.

Sometimes you can learn about clinical trials through advertisements on local radio stations or in the newspaper.

If you might consider traveling to take part in a trial and would like the details about many different arthritis trials, check the Internet. The National Institutes of Health (NIH) has a Web site offering information on more than 4,000 NIH-supported medical studies nationwide (www.clinicaltrials.gov). Another good source of clinical trials on the Web is www.Center-Watch.com.

KEEPING UP WITH RESEARCH

Whether you personally take part in medical research or not, you'll certainly want to know the results of research that is taking place.

Getting the news isn't really that difficult – just open the newspaper, turn on the radio or TV, surf the Internet or ask your doctor. As more people have arthritis and as researchers learn more about it and develop new drugs to treat it, arthritis is a frequent topic discussed in the media.

What is more difficult is finding news that is accurate and putting it into context. It's important that you get your information from reliable sources and scrutinize what you read.

For tips on evaluating the research information you read, see "Identifying Good Research" on page 166.

THE PROGNOSIS FOR LIFE WITH ARTHRITIS

Although no two people and no two cases of arthritis are exactly alike, the odds are that you will live a fulfilling, productive and long life – if you choose to.

While life with a chronic disease holds no certainties, a lot of what happens to you is up to you. Will you take your medications as prescribed? Will you consult your doctor about potential drug reactions or other potential problems? Will you make commitment to exercise and eat healthfully, even when it would be a lot easier not to? Will you take advantage of some of the non-medication techniques that are available to get you through painful times? Will you take an active role in your own health care?

And finally, perhaps the hardest question of all: Will you keep a positive attitude even on days when you feel you have nothing to feel positive about?

Studies show that attitude is an important part of managing arthritis. People who do well tend to recognize the positive aspects of their lives rather than the negatives ones. If you really think about it, you probably will realize that there are a lot of positives in your own life.

Arthritis may change your life, but it doesn't have to control it. While it would be dangerous to deny that you have arthritis and neglect your treatment, it may as harmful in other ways to make arthritis and its treatment the entire focus of your life.

After all, you are still you. If arthritis makes it difficult to do the things you used to do, look for new ways to do them. Or, look for similar activities you can enjoy.

For instance, if you can't hike mountains, perhaps you can enjoy the scenery from the

HOW A DRUG MAKES IT TO MARKET

The American system of new drug approvals, administered by the Food and Drug Administration (FDA), may be the most rigorous in the world. It takes an average of 12 years for a drug to go from development in the lab to the shelves of your local pharmacy – that is, if the drug ever makes it that far. The overwhelming majority never do. In fact, only 1 in 1,000 experimental drugs are ever even tested on people. And of those that do make it to human testing, only 1 in five is eventually approved by the FDA for use by the public.

Here are the steps involved in getting a new drug from the lab to your medicine cabinet:

Preclinical testing. During this stage, which takes approximately three years, a pharmaceutical company conducts laboratory and animal studies to show the biological activity of the compound against the targeted disease. During these tests, the drug is also evaluated for safety.

Investigational New Drug Application (IND). After completing preclinical testing, the company files an investigational new

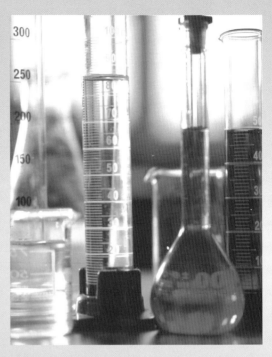

drug application (IND) with the FDA. At this stage, the researchers begin to test the drug on people. The IND becomes effective if the FDA does not disapprove it within 30 days. The IND includes information on results of previous experiments; how, where and by whom new studies will be conducted; the chemical structure of the drug; how the drug

porch of a mountain cabin or enjoy a less strenuous walk through the woods. If arthritis cuts short a college football career, maybe you could pursue a career in coaching or volunteer at your local YMCA. If arthritis in your hands makes it difficult to whip up a gourmet meal from scratch, you can still prepare delicious and nutritious dinners with fresh, pre-cut or frozen vegetables and some help from your local supermarket's deli.

Although having arthritis will never be easy, the prognosis is getting better all the time, with new treatments and new approaches to self-management. With expanding technology as is thought to work in the body; any toxic effects found in animal studies; and how the drug is manufactured. In addition, the IND must be reviewed and approved by the institutional review board where the studies will be conducted, and progress reports on clinical trials must be submitted annually to the FDA.

Phase I clinical trials. This series of tests takes about a year and involves about 20 to 80 healthy volunteers. Researchers study a drug's safety, including the safe dosage range. The studies also determine how a drug is absorbed, distributed, metabolized and excreted, and the duration of its action.

Phase II clinical trials. In this two-year phase, researchers conduct controlled studies of the drug using as many as 100 or more volunteer patients (people with the disease for which the drug was developed) to determine the drug's effectiveness and safety.

Phase III clinical trials. This phase, which lasts about three years, typically involves as many as 1,000 or more patients in participating clinics and hospitals. At this stage, researchers monitor patients closely to determine the drug's effectiveness and to identify any adverse reactions patients may have when taking the drug.

New Drug Application (NDA). If the results of all three phases successfully demonstrate a drug's safety and effectiveness, the company will file a new drug application (NDA) with the FDA. The NDA must include all of the scientific information that the company has gathered. By law the FDA is allowed six months to review the NDA.

Approval. Once the FDA approves the NDA, the new medicine becomes available for physicians to prescribe. The company must continue to submit periodic reports to the FDA, including any reported cases or adverse reactions and appropriate quality-control records. For some medicines, the FDA requires additional studies (Phase IV clinical trials) to evaluate long-term effects.

For more information on how drugs are tested and approved, visit the PhRMA Web site, www.phrma.org./searchcures/new meds/devapprovprocess.phtml

well as the vast array of low-tech things you can do for yourself, you can live a long, fulfilling life despite arthritis. But it's largely up to you.

We hope that *The Arthritis Foundation's Guide To Managing Your Arthritis* has been an informative resource for you as you learn more about arthritis, its treatment and self-management.

Let this book serve as a springboard to learning more about your disease and to incorporating self-management techniques into your daily living. The Arthritis Foundation offers many other resources for educating yourself about arthritis and related conditions, and ways to get involved with your local arthritis community.

CONCLUSION

As you have learned by reading this book, the prognosis for your life with arthritis is full of hope. Proper treatment, including drugs, surgical therapies, exercise and stress reduction methods, can help relieve the pain and other symptoms you experience. Due to recent advances in arthritis drug development, you may be able to slow or halt the damage to your joints in some cases. Never before has your doctor had so many options to counter the effects of arthritis. But the most important leader in your arthritis care and management is you. That's the key message of this book. When you take an active role in managing your arthritis, your overall health and well-being will improve dramatically.

Take the medications your doctor prescribes. Tell him any drug-related problems you experience or supplements you take in addition to your prescription medications. Explore the option of surgery if it is appropriate. Take action steps that will reduce your pain: Exercise, heat and cold treatments, massage therapy, acupuncture, water-exercise classes, weight loss, stress reduction. Refer to the guidelines in this book to help you manage your arthritis, instead of letting your disease manage your life.

Whether you are newly diagnosed with arthritis or have lived with arthritis for years, information is available to help you travel every step of your journey. In addition to this book, the Arthritis Foundation is a great place to begin finding the guidance and support you need. The following section is a brief summary of the many publications, programs and services this organization offers to help people with arthritis take control. With the tools you have from reading this book and the resources of your local Arthritis Foundation chapter, you can manage your arthritis and live a full, abundant life.

Resources

THE ARTHRITIS FOUNDATION

Resources | The Arthritis Foundation

The Arthritis Foundation, the only national, voluntary health organization that works for the more than 43 million Americans with arthritis or related diseases, offers many valuable resources through more than 150 offices nationwide. The chapter that serves your area has information, products, classes and other services to put you in charge of your arthritis. To find the office near you, call 800/283-7800 or search the Arthritis Foundation Web site at www.arthritis.org.

PROGRAMS AND SERVICES

1. Physician referral – Most Arthritis Foundation chapters can provide a list of doctors in your area who specialize in the evaluation and treatment of arthritis and arthritis-related diseases.

2. Exercise programs – The Arthritis Foundation sponsors, develops and coordinates exercise programs for people with arthritis, featuring specially trained instructors. They include:

- JOINT EFFORTS – These classes feature undemanding exercises for all people with arthritis, including those in wheelchairs or walkers.

- PACE* (PEOPLE WITH ARTHRITIS CAN EXERCISE) – These courses feature gentle movements to increase joint flexibility, range of motion, stamina and muscle strength. Accompanying videos are available for home use.

- ARTHRITIS FOUNDATION AQUATIC PROGRAM – These water exercise programs help relieve strain on muscles and joints. An accompanying PEP (Pool Exercise Program) video is

available for home use. This program is also featured in YMCAs nationwide.

3. Educational and Self-Help Courses – The Arthritis Foundation sponsors self-help courses that provide opportunities for discussion and problem-solving among people with arthritis. In addition, the Arthritis Foundation offers courses designed to help people actively manage their particular disease through exercise, medications, relaxation techniques, pain management, nutrition and more. These include the Arthritis Self-Help Course and the Fibromyalgia Self-Help Course.

INFORMATION AND PRODUCTS

Find the latest information about arthritis, including research, medications, government advocacy, programs and services through one of the many information resources offered by the Arthritis Foundation:

1. www.arthritis.org – Information about arthritis is available 24 hours a day on the Internet at the Arthritis Foundation's interactive, comprehensive Web site. Find news about arthritis, ways to get involved, and a variety of self-management and educational products, including books, brochures, videos and more. In addition, the Arthritis Foundation has a new interactive self-management guide for people with arthritis, *Connect and Control: Your Online Arthritis Action Guide.* Via questionnaire responses, Connect and Control helps participants create a customized self-management program for their unique challenges, including tailored information on pain management, joint protection, fitness, diet and more.

2. Arthritis Answers – Call toll-free at 800/283-7800 for 24-hour, automated information about arthritis and Arthritis Foundation resources. Trained volunteers and staff are also available at your local Arthritis Foundation chapter to answer questions or refer you to physicians and other resources. For general questions about arthritis, you can also call 404-872-7100 ext. 1, or e-mail questions to help@arthritis.org.

3. Publications – The Arthritis Foundation offers many publications to educate people with arthritis, as well as their families and friends, about diagnosis, medications, exercise, diet, pain management and more.

- BOOKS – The Arthritis Foundation publishes a variety of books on arthritis to help you

learn to understand and manage your condition, live a healthier life, and cope with the challenges that come with a chronic illness. Order books directly at www.arthritis.org or by calling 800/207-8633. All Arthritis Foundation books are also available at your local bookstore.

- VIDEOS – The Arthritis Foundation produces excellent exercise videos for use in your home or at the pool. To order, call 800/207-8633 or log on to www.arthritis.org.

- BROCHURES – The Arthritis Foundation offers brochures containing concise, understandable information on the many arthritis-related diseases and conditions. Topics include surgery, the latest medications, guidance for working with your doctors and self-managing your illness. Single copies are available free of charge at www.arthritis.org or by calling 800/283-7800.

- *ARTHRITIS TODAY* – This award-winning bi-monthly magazine provides the latest information on research, new treatments, trends and tips from experts and readers to help you manage arthritis. A one-year subscription to *Arthritis Today* is included when you become a member of the Arthritis Foundation. Annual membership is $25 and helps fund research. Call 800/933-0032 for information.

Resources | The Arthritis Foundation

- KIDS GET ARTHRITIS TOO – This newsletter focusing on juvenile rheumatic diseases is published six times a year. Features speak to children and teens with the illness as well as to their parents. Stories examine the latest news in diagnosis, treatment and research of children's rheumatic diseases, as well as helpful ways kids can cope with their illnesses and the challenges they bring. This newsletter is now a benefit of membership in the Arthritis Foundation and can be ordered for free. Call 800/283-7800 for information.

RESEARCH AND ADVOCACY

The Arthritis Foundation is the second-largest funding source for arthritis research, behind the National Institutes of Health (NIH). In the year 2000, the Foundation funded more than $24 million in both basic and clinical research targeted at better understanding various forms of arthritis and related conditions and improving treatment for people with them.

The Arthritis Foundation is also involved in numerous advocacy issues, from working to increase funding for arthritis research by the federal government to ensuring access to care.

To learn how you can be advocate for people with arthritis and play a role in forming public policy, call your local Arthritis Foundation office or log on to www.arthritis.org.

Glossary & Index

MANAGING YOUR ARTHRITIS

Glossary

A

ACUPUNCTURE – Eastern medicine technique in which thin needles are used to puncture the body at specific sites along energy pathways call meridians. Although still widely considered an alternative therapy, acupuncture is gaining acceptance in Western medicine, primarily for use in pain relief. Acupressure is another form of this treatment, but one involving hand pressure rather than needle punctures.

ACUTE ILLNESS – An illness of short duration that comes on quickly and produces severe symptoms.

AMERICAN COLLEGE OF RHEUMA-TOLOGY (ACR) – Organization that provides a professional, educational and research forum for rheumatologists across the country. Among its functions are helping determine what symptoms and signs define the various types of rheumatic disease diagnoses and what the appropriate treatments are for those diagnoses.

AMERICAN ACADEMY OF ORTHOPAEDIC SURGEONS – Organization that provides education and practice management services for orthopaedic surgeons and allied health professionals. The Academy also serves as an advocate for improved patient care and informs the public about the science of orthopaedics.

ANALGESIC – A type of medication used to treat pain.

ANESTHESIA – The induction of partial or complete loss of sensation. Used to perform surgery and other medical procedures.

ANKYLOSING SPONDYLITIS (AS) – A form of arthritis that mainly affects the spine and sacroiliac joints (where the spine attaches to the pelvis). In severe cases, AS may cause the spine to become fused and rigid.

ANTINUCLEAR ANTIBODIES (ANA) – Proteins produced by the immune system against the cell nucleus (control center). They are often present in people with certain forms of the arthritis, including lupus and scleroderma. A test showing a positive ANA can help a doctor in diagnosis.

ASSOCIATION OF RHEUMATOLOGY HEALTH PROFESSIONALS – A division of the American College of Rheumatology comprised of health professionals – including nurses, physical and occupational therapists, psychologists, pharmacists, dietitians, epidemiologists and others – who work with people with arthritis-related diseases and/or study those diseases.

ARTHRODESIS – A surgical procedure in which the two bones that form a joint are fused into a single, immovable unit.

ARTHROPLASTY – Also called joint replacement surgery, a procedure in which a damaged joint is surgically removed and replaced with a synthetic one.

ARTHROSCOPY – A surgical procedure in which a thin, lighted scope is inserted into the joint through a small incision or puncture site, allowing the joint's interior to be viewed on a monitor. Through additional small incisions, tools can be inserted to do minor surgical repairs such as smoothing rough cartilage or removing cartilage fragments.

ASPIRATION – The withdrawal of fluid from the body, such as synovial fluid from the joint.

AUTOIMMUNE DISEASE – A disease in which the immune system, which is designed to protect the body from foreign invaders such as viruses and bacteria, instead turns against the body and causes damage to the body's healthy tissue.

B

BIOFEEDBACK – The use of electronic instruments to measure body functions and feed that information back to you, allowing you to learn how to control body processes, such as heart rate or blood pressure, that are generally thought to be out of conscious control.

BIOLOGIC FIXATION – A process by which joint prostheses with specially designed, porous surfaces are held in place by the growth of patients' own bone into the prostheses.

BIOLOGIC RESPONSE MODIFIERS – Drugs that target and modify specific pathways involved in the development of disease. The current biologic response modifiers used for rheumatoid arthritis target specific immune system chemicals, called cytokines, that play a role in the inflammation and damage of the disease, while leaving other immune-system components intact.

BIOPSY – A procedure to remove a piece of tissue for study. Depending on the piece of tissue examined, your doctor may use a biopsy to diagnose diseases of the joint, muscle, skin or blood vessels.

Glossary

BISPHOSPHONATES – A class of medications that inhibit bone resorption (see below) and are used to treat bone diseases such as osteoporosis.

BONE RESORPTION – The loss of bone through physiological means. In the body, existing bone is constantly being resorbed while new bone grows to take its place. Bone resorption is essential to healthy bones unless it outpaces the growth of new bone.

BONE FUSION – The growth of two bones into a solid, immobile unit. Surgeons often promote bone fusion by removing the cartilage from two bones at a joint and then holding them in place by a cast, splint or pins until the bones grow together. Joint fusion offers pain relief for joints that typically aren't replaced with prostheses.

BOUCHARD'S NODES – Knobby growths of bone that commonly appear on the middle knuckle in people with osteoarthritis.

BURSAE – Small, fluid-filled sacs that cushion and lubricate joints.

BURSITIS – Inflammation of the bursae (fluid-filled sacs that lubricate the joints), which can cause pain, tenderness and stiffness of the nearby joint.

C

CAPSAICIN – A pain-relieving substance derived from cayenne pepper that is the active ingredient in some analgesic rubs.

CARPAL TUNNEL SYNDROME – Compression of the median nerve, which supplies the thumbside of the hand as it enters the palm. Often caused by inflammation in the carpal tunnel, the space between bones of the wrist through which the nerve and tendons run, it can cause numbness of the middle and index finger and weakness of the thumb.

CARTILAGE – A smooth, rubbery tissue that covers the ends of the bones at the joints and acts as a shock absorber, allowing the joint to move smoothly.

CHIROPRACTIC – Practice of healing based on spinal manipulation and the belief that illness stems from malalignment of the spinal cord.

CHRONIC ILLNESS – An illness of long duration, possibly a lifetime.

COLLAGEN – A protein that is the primary component of cartilage and other connective tissue.

COMPLEMENT – A protein in the blood involved in certain forms of inflammation. Complement levels are often low in people with systemic lupus erythematosus, for example.

COX-2 SPECIFIC INHIBITOR – A type of nonsteroidal anti-inflammatory drug (NSAID) that is designed to be safer for the stomach than other NSAIDs. COX-2 inhibitors work by inhibiting hormone-like substances in the body that cause pain and inflammation without interfering with similar substances that protect the stomach lining.

CYTOKINES – Chemical messengers in the body that play a role in the immune response.

D

DERMATOMYOSITIS – The disease in which generally muscle weakness is accompanied by a skin rash (see Polymyositis).

DEXA – Short for dual-energy X-ray absorptiometry, a scan that measures bone density at the hip and spine to diagnose osteoporosis and evaluate bone density.

DMARDS – Short for disease-modifying antirheumatic drugs, a class of medications that work to modify the course of rheumatoid arthritis and other forms of inflammatory arthritis, slowing or even stopping its progression.

E

EPIDURAL ANESTHESIA – Anesthetic injected directly into the spinal canal, between the spinal column and the outermost cover of the spinal cord. Epidural anesthesia is used to numb the lower half of the body and is often used in knee surgery.

EROSIONS – A wearing away of the bone in the joint caused by inflammation of the joint lining.

ERYTHROCYTE SEDIMENTATION RATE (ESR) – Also referred to as sed rate, a test measuring how fast red blood cells (erythrocytes) clump together and fall to the bottom of a test tube like sediment. A high (fast) sedimentation rate signals the presence of inflammation, possibly indicating an inflammatory disease such as rheumatoid arthritis.

Glossary

F

FATIGUE – A generalized, long-lasting feeling of tiredness or sleepiness that isn't relieved by sleep or rest.

FIBROMYALGIA – A syndrome characterized by widespread muscle pain, the presence of tender points (or points on the body that feel painful on pressure) and often debilitating fatigue and other symptoms.

G

GLUCOCORTICOIDS – A group of hormones, including cortisol, produced by the adrenal glands. They can be synthetically produced (that is, made in a laboratory) and have powerful anti-inflammatory effects. They are sometimes called corticosteroids or steroids.

GOUT – A form of arthritis that occurs when uric acid builds up in the blood and deposits as crystals in the joints and other tissue. A joint, such as the big toe, affected by gout may be excruciatingly painful, and shiny and purplish in appearance.

H

HAMMER TOES – Toes that are dislocated and look like the hammers in a piano. The problem is often seen in people with RA and results in ulcers on the tops of the toes and pain when walking.

HEBERDEN'S NODES – Knobby growths of bone that may appear on the knuckles nearest the nails in people with osteoarthritis.

HYALURONIC ACID – A substance in the synovial fluid of the joints that give the fluid its viscosity and shock-absorbing properties.

I

IMMUNE SYSTEM – The body's natural system of defense against invaders, such as viruses and bacteria, that it sees as harmful.

INFECTIOUS ARTHRITIS – A form of arthritis that occurs when a blood-borne infection settles in a joint or joints.

INFLAMMATION – An immune-system response to injury or infection that causes heat, redness and swelling in the affected area. In some forms of arthritis, joint and organ inflammation occurs as a result of a faulty immune response to the body's own tissues.

INTERNIST – A doctor who specializes in the diagnosis, prevention and treatment of all forms of adult disease. Training for an internist requires four years of medical school, followed by a three-year in-hospital residency. Internists may choose to take additional subspecialty training in fields such as rheumatology, endocrinology, cardiology or gastroenterology.

J

JOINT – The juncture of two or more bones in the body. The human body contains more than 150 joints, some of which are rigid and others that allow the body to move in many different positions.

JUVENILE RHEUMATOID ARTHRITIS – A type of arthritis that occurs in children under age 16. There are three different forms of JRA, differentiated primarily by the number of joints they affect.

L

LIGAMENTS – Tough bands of connective tissue that attach bones to bones and help keep them together at a joint.

LUPUS – A term often used to refer to systemic lupus erythematosus, an autoimmune disease that can affect the joints, skin, blood, lungs, kidneys, and cardiovascular and nervous systems.

M

MRI – Short for magnetic resonance imaging, MRI is a procedure in which a very strong magnet is used to pass a force through the body to create a clear, detailed image of a cross-section of the body.

MUSCLE – Fibrous tissue in the body holds us upright and gives the body movement, including both movement that we consciously initiate (such as waving a hand) and movement of which we are scarcely aware (such movement of the blood through the vessels or food through the digestive system).

N

NARCOTIC – A drug used to relieve severe pain by depressing brain function. The name is used particularly for morphine and other derivatives of opium.

NONSTEROIDAL ANTI-INFLAMMATORY DRUGS (NSAIDS) – A class of medications commonly used to ease

Glossary

the pain and inflammation of many forms of arthritis.

NURSE AND NURSE PRACTITIONER – A person who has received education and training in health care, particularly patient care. Many nurses have earned a registered nurse degree, noted by an RN in their title. Nurse practitioners are registered nurses with advanced training and emphasis in primary care, who can diagnose illness and, in many states, prescribe medication.

O

OCCUPATIONAL THERAPIST (OT) – A licensed health-care professional who is trained to evaluate the impact of arthritis on daily activities. OTs can help devise easier ways to perform activities that put less stress on fragile joints and can prescribe splints and assistive devices.

ORTHOPAEDIC SURGEON – A doctor who specializes in surgery involving the musculoskeletal system, including the bones and joints

ORTHOTIST – A paramedical health professional who designs, fabricates and fits orthotic devices, such as splints, braces and shoe inserts, to help people function better.

OSTEOARTHRITIS (OA) – The most common form of arthritis. OA causes cartilage breakdown at certain joints (including the spine, hands, hips and knees) resulting in pain and deformity.

OSTEOPOROSIS – A condition in which the body loses so much bone mass that bones are susceptible to disabling fractures under the slightest trauma.

OSTEOTOMY – A surgical procedure that involves cutting and repositioning a bone, usually performed in cases of severe joint malalignment.

P

PEDIATRIC RHEUMATOLOGIST – A doctor who specializes in treating arthritis and related conditions in children.

PHYSICAL THERAPIST (PT) – A licensed health-care professional who specializes in using exercise to treat medical conditions. A PT may prescribe canes and splints and some are trained in massage.

PLACEBO EFFECT – The phenomenon in which a person receiving an inactive drug or therapy experiences a reduction in symptoms.

PODAGRA – Inflammation of the foot, particularly the big toe, caused by gout, a form of arthritis that occurs when uric acid builds up in the blood and deposits as crystals in the joints and other tissue.

POLYMYALGIA RHEUMATICA – A disease causing joint and muscle pain in the neck, shoulders and hips and a general feeling of malaise. The disease is usually marked by a high sedimentation rate (see erythrocyte sedimentation rate) and occasionally by a fever.

POLYMYOSITIS – An arthritis-related disease in which generalized weakness results from inflammation of the muscles, primarily those of the shoulders, upper arms, thighs and hips. When muscle weakness is accompanied by a skin rash, the diagnosis is dermatomyositis.

PROSTAGLANDINS – Hormonelike substances in the body that play a role in pain and inflammation among other body functions.

PROTEIN A IMMUNOADSORPTION THERAPY – A treatment for rheumatoid arthritis that involves filtering the blood plasma through a special column to remove antibodies associated with RA.

PSORIATIC ARTHRITIS – A form of arthritis that is accompanied by the skin disease psoriasis

Q

QI GONG – An Asian practice that incorporates meditation, breathing exercises and movement to promote health and self-healing.

R

RANGE OF MOTION – The distance and angles at which your joints can be moved, extended and rotated in various directions.

RAYNAUD'S PHENOMENON – A condition in which the blood vessels in the hands go into spasms in response to stress or cold temperatures, resulting in pain, tingling and numbness.

RESECTION – A surgical procedure that involves removing all or part of a bone, sometimes used to relieve joint pain and stiffness.

REVISION – A second or subsequent surgery done to correct problems with a joint prosthesis that has broken, loosened or become infected.

Glossary

RHEUMATIC DISEASE – A general term referring to conditions characterized by pain and stiffness of the joints or muscles. The American College of Rheumatology currently recognizes more than 100 rheumatic diseases. The term is often used interchangeably with "arthritis" (meaning joint inflammation), but not all rheumatic diseases affect the joints or involve inflammation.

RHEUMATISM – A term used loosely (thought not as widely used as it was in the past) to refer to conditions that cause pain and swelling in the joints and supporting tissues.

RHEUMATOID ARTHRITIS – A chronic inflammatory form of arthritis in which the body's otherwise protective immune system turns against the body and attacks tissues of the joints, causing pain, inflammation and deformity.

RHEUMATOID FACTOR (RF) – A blood protein (antibody) that is found in high levels in many people with rheumatoid arthritis. It is often associated with RA severity or disease activity, and its presence can be helpful to a doctor in making a diagnosis.

RHEUMATOLOGIST – A doctor who specializes in treating arthritis and related diseases. Rheumatologists typically spend three years beyond medical school in an internal medicine residency and then spend an additional two to three years of clinical training in the diagnosis and treatment of arthritis.

RISK/BENEFIT RATIO – The comparison of a treatment's risk of causing adverse effects (and the severity of those effects) to the treatment's potential benefit to the patient. Risks and benefits must be weighed for all treatments a person is considering.

S

SACROILIAC – The joints where the spine attaches to the pelvis.

SALICYLATES – A subcategory of nonsteroidal anti-inflammatory drugs (NSAIDs), which includes aspirin. Also describes topical creams containing salicylic acid that relieve pain and inflammation.

SCLERODERMA – An umbrella term for several diseases that involve the abnormal growth of connective tissue. In most cases, the effects of this overgrowth are limited to the skin and underlying tissues, but in others, tissue overgrowth can affect the joints, blood vessels and internal organs.

SED RATE – See erythrocyte sedimentation rate.

SERMS (SELECTIVE ESTROGEN RECEPTOR MOLECULES) – A class of medications that work much like estrogen to slow bone loss, but lack estrogen's side effects on uterine and breast tissues.

SEROSITIS – Inflammation of the lining of some of the organs such as the heart and lungs

SJÖGREN'S SYNDROME – An arthritis-related disease in which the immune system attacks moisture-producing glands of the body, causing dryness of the eyes, mouth and vagina.

SPLINT – Devices made from metal, plastic, cloth or moldable foam that are used to support or stabilize a joint or to position a joint in a way that prevents further irritation or injury to joint or soft tissues surrounding it

SPONDYLARTHROPATHIES – A group of arthritis-related diseases that primarily affect the spine.

STEM CELLS – Progenitor cells in the body that have the ability to differentiate into different cells. Some experimental therapies for some autoimmune diseases involve removing stem cells from the body and freezing; destroying damaging cells; and then reinfusing healthy stem cells back into the body to regrow and replace the damaging cells that were destroyed.

SYNOVECTOMY – Surgical removal of a diseased joint lining (see synovium).

SYNOVIAL FLUID – A slippery liquid secreted by the synovium that lubricates the joint, making movement easier.

SYNOVIUM – A thin membrane that lines the joint capsule and can become inflamed in rheumatoid arthritis.

SYSTEMIC – A term used to refer to anything, such as a disease or medication, that affects the whole body. Rheumatoid arthritis, for example, is a systemic disease.

T

TAI CHI – An ancient Chinese practice that involves gentle, fluid movements and meditation to help strengthen muscles, improve balance and relieve stress

Glossary

TENDER POINTS – Specific, precise areas on the body that are particularly painful upon the application of slight pressure. The finding of tender points is useful in the diagnosis of fibromyalgia.

TENDINITIS – Painful inflammation of a tendon often caused by injury or overuse, and less frequently by infection or a form of arthritis such as rheumatoid arthritis or ankylosing spondylitis.

TENDONS – Thick connective tissue that attaches the muscles to the bones.

TENS – A treatment for pain that uses a small device to direct mild electric pulses to nerves in the painful area.

TUMOR NECROSIS FACTOR (TNF) – A cytokine (chemical messenger) in the body that plays a role in inflammation and tissue destruction in diseases such as rheumatoid arthritis, but also is important for normal function of the immune system. Blocking TNF with biologically derived drugs has proven to ease symptoms and inhibit joint destruction in RA.

U

URIC ACID – A bodily waste product that is excreted through the kidneys. When the body produces too much uric acid or doesn't excrete it efficiently, excess uric acid can deposit as crystals in the joint and other tissues, a condition known as gout (see Gout).

URINALYSIS – The analysis of urine using physical, chemical and microscopic tests to detect the presence of infection, levels or uric acid excreted or abnormal constituents.

V

VASCULITIS – Inflammation of the blood vessels that can be a complication of some forms of inflammatory forms of arthritis and related conditions.

VISCOSUPPLEMENTS – Products injected into osteoarthritis joints to replace hyaluronic acid that usually gives the joint fluid its viscosity. This process is known as viscosupplementation. Viscosupplements are currently approved only for OA of the knee, but are being tested on other joints.

Y

YOGA – An ancient Indian practice that involves a series of body postures and includes exercise, meditation and breathing components to improve posture and balance and help relieve stress on the joints, as well as emotional stress.

Index

Index

Index

Index

H

H2 blockers, 63
Hammer toes, 182
Head tilts (exercise), 119
Head turns (exercise), 118
Health-care provider, as information source, 44
Health-care team, members of, 38–42
Heat treatments, 135–136
Heberden's nodes, 15, 182
Hexadrol. See Dexamethasone
Hinge joints, 9
Hip turns (exercise), 126
Histamine blockers, 63
HLA-DR4, as indication of rheumatic arthritis, 16, 31
HLBA-B27, as indication of ankylosing spondylitis, 18, 19, 31
Hormones, 68
 role of, in rheumatoid arthritis, 16–17
Hyalgan. See Hyaluronate sodium
Hyaluronate sodium, 78, 90
Hyaluronic acid, 182
Hydrocet. See Hydrocodone with acetaminophen
Hydrocodone, 65
 with acetaminophen, 77
Hydrocortisone, 79
Hydrocortone. See Hydrocortisone
Hydroxychloroquine sulfate, 66–67, 81, 88
Hylan G-F 20, 78, 90

I

Ibuprofen, 53, 60, 74
Icy Hot, 64, 78
IL-1ra, 163
Imaging tests, 31–33
 DEXA scans, 32
 magnetic resonance imaging, 32
 ultrasonography, 32–33
 X-rays, 31–32
Immune system, 182
Imuran. See Azathioprine

Indocin. See Indomethacin
Indomethacin, 74
Indocin SR. See Indomethacin
Infectious arthritis, 22, 182
 diagnosis of, 31
 factors in development of, 22
Inflammation, 182
Inflammatory bowel disease, 30
Infliximab, 67, 80
Information
 getting drug, 70, 72
 sources of, 42–47
Injectable gold, 82
Interleukin-1 (IL-1), 67
Internist, 182
Investigational New Drug Application (IND), 168
Isometric exercises, 116–117
Interleukin-1 receptor antagonist (IL-1ra), 163

J

Joint alignment, congenital abnormalities in, 15–16
Joint dislocation, 111
Joint fluid exam, 31
Joint protection, 134–135
Joints, 182
 ball-and-socket, 9
 defined, 8, 9
 hinge, 9
 normal, 8
 with osteoarthritis, 8
 overuse of, 16
 sacroiliac, 18
Journal, keeping, in stress reduction, 148–149
Juvenile arthritis, 17
 diagnosis of, 30
Juvenile rheumatoid arthritis, 16, 17, 182
 diagnosis of, 30
 statistics on, 17

K

Kava kava, 156
Ketoprofen, 53, 74
Kidney, biopsy of, 33
Kineret. See Anakinra
Knee extension (exercise), 130

L

Lab tests, 29–31
 anti-DNA, 30–31
 antinuclear antibody, 30
 complement, 31
 complete blood count, 30
C-reactive protein, 30
 erthrocyte sedimentation rate, 29–30
 joint fluid exam, 31
Lyme serology, 31
 rheumatoid factor, 30
 tissue typing, 31
 uric acid, 30
 urinalysis, 30
Lansoprazole, 63
Leflunomide, 66, 81, 89
Leukotriene synthesis, 154
Ligaments, 9, 182
Local anesthesia, 100
Lodine. See Etodolac
Lodine XL. See Etodolac
Loosening, of the prosthesis, 111
Lopurin. See Allopurinol
Lorcet. See Hydrocodone with acetaminophen
Lortab. See Hydrocodone with acetaminophen
Ludiomil. See Maprotiline
Lupus, 19–20, 182
 association with Raynaud's phenomenon, 23
 diagnosis of, 30, 31, 32, 33, 34
 environmental factors in, 20
 gender as factor in, 19
 genetics and, 20
 melatonin and, 156
 statistics on, 19

Index

Index

Index

S

Sacroiliac joints, 18, 184
S-adenosylmethionine, 156
Salflex. See Salsalate
Salicylates, 64, 78, 184
Salsalate, 75
Salsitab. See Salsalate
SAM-e, 156
Sandimmune. See Cyclosporine
Scleroderma, 22, 184
    association with Raynaud's
       phenomenon, 23
    diagnosis of, 30, 34
Scleroderma Foundation, 46
SED rate, 184
Selective estrogen receptor molecules
    (SERMs), 68, 184
Selective serotonin reuptake inhibitors
    (SSRIs), 69, 82, 83–84
Self back rub (exercise), 120
Self-management, 2–3
Self-massage, 137
Sertraline, 69, 84
Shoulder circles (exercise), 119
Shoulder rotation (exercise), 121
Shoulder shrugs (exercise), 119
Side bends (exercise), 124
Side leg kick (exercise), 126
Sinequan. See Doxepin
Sjögren's syndrome, 22, 184
    as autoimmune disease, 22
    diagnosis of, 30
    need for dentist and, 41
Skier's squat (exercise), 127
Skin, biopsy of, 33
Social worker, 40
Sodium salicylate, 76
Solganol, 82
Sonata. See Zaleplon
Spinal stenosis, 23–24
    diagnosis of, 32
Splints, 133–134, 184
Spondyloarthropathies, 184
    ankylosing spondylitis as, 18
    diagnosis of, 31

Sportscreme, 64
Stem cells, 184
Stem cell transplantation, 163–165
Sterapred. See Prednisone
Stomach distress, NSAIDs in, 62–63
Stress diary, keeping, 144–145
Stress reduction, 140, 144–149
    biofeedback in, 147–149
    keeping journal in, 148–149
    keeping stress diary in, 144–145
    relaxation exercises in, 146–147
    relaxation techniques in, 145–146
Sulfasalazine, 82, 89
Sulfinpyrazone, 70, 85
Sulindac, 76
Supartz. See Hyaluronate sodium
Support hose, 98
Surgery, 94–101
    anesthesia for, 100–101
    arthrodesis, 95
    arthroplasty or total joint
      replacement, 95–96
    arthroscopy, 96
    infection from, 110–111
    as option, 97–100
    osteotomy, 94–95
    questions to ask doctor about,
      102–103
    resection, 95
    risks and prevention, 110–111
    synovectomy, 94
Swedish massage, 137–138
Synovectomy, 34, 94, 96, 184
Synovial fluid, 9, 184
Synovium, 9, 184
    assessing inflammation of, 33
    biopsy of, 33
    inflammation of, 16
Synvisc. See Hylan G-F 20
Systemic, 184
Systemic lupus erythematosus (SLE).
See Lupus

T

Tagamet. See Cimetidine

Tai chi, 131, 184
Temazepam, 69, 84
Temporal artery, biopsy of, 33
Temporal arthritis, diagnosis of, 33
Temporomendibular joint disorder,
    18, 41
Tender points, 185
    in fibromyalgia, 17, 28, 35
Tendinitis, 185
Tendons, 9, 185
TENS (transcutaneous electrical nerve
    stimulation), 140, 185
Therapeutic Mineral Ice, 64, 78
Thigh firmer and knee stretch
    (exercise), 129
Thumb bend and finger curl
    (exercise), 123
Tiptoe (exercise), 127
Tissue typing, 31
Tolectin. See Tolmetin sodium
Tolmetin sodium, 76
Topical analgesics, 64, 78
Total joint replacement, 95–96
Tramadol, 63, 65, 77
Transcutaneous electrical nerve
    stimulation (TENS), 140, 185
Trazodone, 84
Trazon. See Trazodone
Treatment, getting proper, 38–42
Trexall. See Methotrexate
Trialodine. See Trazodone
Triamcinolone, 80
Tricosal. See Choline and magnesium
    salicylates
Tricyclics, 65, 69, 82, 83
Trigger point therapy, 138
Trilisate. See Choline and magnesium
    salicylates
Trunk twist (exercise), 124
Tumor necrosis factor (TNF), 67, 185
Tylenol. See Acetaminophen
Tylenol with codeine. See Aceta
    minophen with codeine
Type II collagen, 10, 15

Index

U

Ulcer risk, nonsteroidal anti-inflammatory drugs as, 61
Ultram. See Tramadol
Ultrasonography, 32–33
Uric acid, 185
    buildup of, in gout, 19, 30, 138
Urinalysis, 30, 185

V

Vasculitis, 24, 185
    diagnosis of, 30, 31, 33
Vicodin. See Hydrocodone with acetaminophen
Vioxx. See Rofecoxib
Viral-related aarthritis, 22
Viscosupplements, 78, 90, 185

Visualization, 146
Vitamin D
    daily requirement for, 71
    supplements, 68
Voltaren. See Diclofenac sodium

W

Water exercise program, 132
Water therapy, 136–137
Weight, controlling, 134–135, 138–140
Weight loss, 138–140
Wrist bend (exercise), 123
Wygesic. See Propoxyphene hydrochloride

X

X-rays, 31–32

Y

Yoga, 131, 185

Z

Zaleplon, 69
Zantac. See Ranitidine hydrochloride
Zoloft. See Sertraline
Zolpidem, 69, 85
ZORprin. See Aspirin
Zostrix. See Capsaicin
Zostrix HP. See Capsaicin
Zyloprim. See Allopurinol